Self-Assessment C

Veterinary Dentistry

2nd Edition

Self-Assessment Color Review

Veterinary Dentistry

2nd Edition

Edited by

Frank JM Verstraete
DrMedVet, BVSc (Hons), MMedVet, Dipl AVDC, Dipl ECVS, Dipl EVDC
University of California – Davis
Davis, California, USA

Anson J Tsugawa
VMD, Dipl AVDC
Dog and Cat Dentist, Inc.
Culver City, California, USA

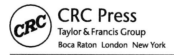

CRC Press
Taylor & Francis Group
Boca Raton London New York

CRC Press is an imprint of the
Taylor & Francis Group, an **informa** business

CRC Press
Taylor & Francis Group
6000 Broken Sound Parkway NW, Suite 300
Boca Raton, FL 33487-2742

Printed on acid-free paper
Version Date: 20150805

International Standard Book Number-13: 978-1-4822-2545-7 (Paperback)

This book contains information obtained from authentic and highly regarded sources. While all reasonable efforts have been made to publish reliable data and information, neither the author[s] nor the publisher can accept any legal responsibility or liability for any errors or omissions that may be made. The publishers wish to make clear that any views or opinions expressed in this book by individual editors, authors or contributors are personal to them and do not necessarily reflect the views/opinions of the publishers. The information or guidance contained in this book is intended for use by medical, scientific or health-care professionals and is provided strictly as a supplement to the medical or other professional's own judgement, their knowledge of the patient's medical history, relevant manufacturer's instructions and the appropriate best practice guidelines. Because of the rapid advances in medical science, any information or advice on dosages, procedures or diagnoses should be independently verified. The reader is strongly urged to consult the relevant national drug formulary and the drug companies' and device or material manufacturers' printed instructions, and their websites, before administering or utilizing any of the drugs, devices or materials mentioned in this book. This book does not indicate whether a particular treatment is appropriate or suitable for a particular individual. Ultimately it is the sole responsibility of the medical professional to make his or her own professional judgements, so as to advise and treat patients appropriately. The authors and publishers have also attempted to trace the copyright holders of all material reproduced in this publication and apologize to copyright holders if permission to publish in this form has not been obtained. If any copyright material has not been acknowledged please write and let us know so we may rectify in any future reprint.

Visit the Taylor & Francis Web site at
http://www.taylorandfrancis.com

and the CRC Press Web site at
http://www.crcpress.com

Preface

We hope that the contents of this book will be a true reflection of its title. This text was written to give you, the reader, whether you are a keen final-year student, a resident, a practitioner, or a board-certified specialist, an opportunity to assess your knowledge of veterinary dentistry, based on a series of well-illustrated questions. Hopefully, it will stimulate your interest and promote further study. The book should be used in combination with standard dentistry textbooks; it is not intended to substitute for any of them, and by no means should this book be seen as a stand-alone volume. If, at the end of an evening, having gone through a few questions, you find your desk covered with half a dozen opened veterinary and human dental textbooks, and several article reprints scattered in between, we will have achieved our goal!

Care has been taken to ensure that the material presented is informative and factually correct. However, the format of the book does not allow in-depth discussion of the various nuances that may exist and be applicable to a clinical case. Equally, the random nature of the questions and the limited volume of this book do not allow a systematic and comprehensive review of the subject matter. Although we recognize these shortcomings, we urge the reader to see beyond the limitations of the format and use this book for its intended purpose of self-assessment.

Frank JM Verstraete
Anson J Tsugawa

Acknowledgements

We are indebted to all the authors who have contributed to the first edition of this book:

David A Crossley BVetMed, PhD, MRCVS, Dipl EVDC
Linda J DeBowes DVM, MS, Dipl ACVIM, Dipl AVDC
Gregg A DuPont DVM, Dipl AVDC
Edward R Eisner AB, DVM, Dipl AVDC
Peter P Emily DDS
Peter Fahrenkrug DrMedVet, DrMedDent, Dipl EVDC
Patricia Frost DVM, Dipl AVDC
Cecilia Gorrel BSc, MA, Vet MB, DDS, MRCVS, Dipl EVDC
T Keith Grove DDS, MS, VMD, Dipl AVDC, Dipl ABP
Colin E Harvey BVSc, FRCVS, Dipl ACVS, Dipl AVDC, Dipl EVDC
Philippe Hennet DV, Dipl AVDC, Dipl EVDC
Steven E Holmstrom DVM, Dipl AVDC
J Geoffrey Lane BVetMed, FRCVS
Kenneth F Lyon DVM, Dipl AVDC
Sandra Manfra Marretta DVM, Dipl ACVS, Dipl AVDC
W Leon Scrutchfield DVM, Dipl ACVIM
Andries W van Foreest DrMedVet
Chris J Visser BVSc, DVM, MRCVS, Dipl AVDC, Dipl EVDC

We thank Travis J Henry DVM for contributing the equine questions for the second edition.

Picture acknowledgements

8 Photograph **8b** reproduced with permission from Nemec A, Daniaux L, Johnson E, Peralta S, Verstraete FJM (2014). Craniomaxillofacial abnormalities in dogs with congenital palatal defects: computed tomographic findings. *Veterinary Surgery*, doi: 10.1111/j.1532–950X.2014.12129.x. [Epub ahead of print].

12 Illustration **12b** reprinted with permission of the American Veterinary Dental College - http://www.avdc.org/nomenclature.html (accessed 01/17/2015).

21 Photograph reproduced with permission from Rusbridge C, Heath S, Gunn-Moore DA, Knowler SP, Johnston N, McFadyen AK (2010). Feline orofacial pain syndrome (FOPS): a retrospective study of 113 cases. *Journal of Feline Medicine and Surgery*, 12:498–508.

23 Photograph **23a** courtesy of Dr Helena Kuntsi-Vaattovaara, Veikkola, Finland; photograph **23b** courtesy of Dr Tony Woodward, Colorado Springs, CO, USA.

31 Illustrations **31a** and **31b** reproduced with permission from Luotonen N, Kuntsi-Vaattovaara H, Sarkiala-Kessel E, Junnila JJ, Laitinen-Vapaavuori O, Verstraete FJM (2014). Vital pulp therapy in dogs: 190 cases (2001–2011). *Journal of the American Veterinary Medical Association*, 244:449–59.

39, 68, 174, 200a Illustrations courtesy of Hu-Friedy Mfg. Co., Chicago, USA.

42 Photograph courtesy of Ms Julie Averill-Martin, Averill Maine Coon Cats, Sacramento, CA, USA.

46 Photograph courtesy of Drs Paul Simoens and Jan Declercq, University of Ghent, Belgium.

51 Photograph reprinted with permission from Verstraete FJM (1993). Dental pathology and microbiology. In DG Slatter (ed) *Textbook of Small Animal Surgery* (2nd edn), WB Saunders, Philadelphia, USA.

58 Photographs **58c** and **58d** reproduced with permission from Bar-Am Y, Verstraete FJM (2010). Elastic training for the prevention of mandibular drift following mandibulectomy in dogs: 18 cases (2005–2008). *Veterinary Surgery*, 39:574–80.

75, 127, 178, 226 Photographs reproduced with permission from van Foreest AW (1996). Verkleuring van gebitselementen bij gezelschapsdieren. *Tijdschrift voor Diergeneeskunde*, 121(11):316–22.

94 Photograph **94a** reproduced with permission from van Foreest AW (1996). Verkleuring van gebitselementen bij gezelschapsdieren. *Tijdschrift voor Diergeneeskunde*, 121(11):316–22. Photograph **94b** reproduced with permission from Verstraete FJM, Ligthelm AJ (1992). Dental trauma caused by internal fixation of mandibular osteotomies in the dog. *Journal of Veterinary and Comparative Orthopaedics and Traumatology*, 5:104–108.

95 Illustrations accompanying the answer were redrawn from Shillingburg HT, Jacobi R, Brackett SE (1987). *Fundamentals of Tooth Preparations for Cast Metal and Porcelain Restorations.* Quintessence Publishing Co., Chicago.

98 Photograph reprinted with permission from Verstraete FJM (1993). Behandeling van orale tumoren bij de hond. *Vlaams Diergeneeskundig Tijdschrift,* **62**:143–50.

99 Photographs **99a** and **99b** reproduced with permission from Verstraete FJM, Arzi B, Huey DJ, Cissell DD, Athanasiou KA (2014). Regenerating mandibular bone using rhBMP-2: part 2 - treatment of chronic, defect non-union fractures. *Veterinary Surgery,* doi: 10.1111/j.1532-950X.2014.12122.x. [Epub ahead of print].

110 Micrograph reproduced courtesy of Dr Bjorn Klinge, Karolinska Institute, Stockholm, Sweden.

115 Illustration **115c** reproduced with permission from Tsugawa AJ, Lommer MJ, Verstraete FJM (2012). Extraction of canine teeth in dogs. In FJM Verstraete and MJ Lommer (eds) *Oral and Maxillofacial Surgery in Dogs and Cats* (1st edn), Saunders–Elsevier, Edinburgh, UK.

122 Photograph **122a** reproduced with permission from Verstraete FJM, Osofsky A (2005). Dentistry in pet rabbits. *Compendium on Continuing Education for the Practicing Veterinarian,* **27**:671–84.

123 Photograph **123a** courtesy of Halimeter®, Simi Valley, CA, USA.

124 Photograph **124a** courtesy of Piezosurgery® Inc., Columbus, OH, USA.

146 Photographs **146a** and **146b** reproduced with permission from Verstraete FJM, Osofsky A (2005). Dentistry in pet rabbits. *Compendium on Continuing Education for the Practicing Veterinarian,* **27**:671–84.

151 Photograph **151b** courtesy of iM3, Inc., Vancouver, WA, USA.

154 Illustration reproduced with permission from Peeters MJ (2012). Principles of salivary gland surgery. In FJM Verstraete and MJ Lommer (eds) *Oral and Maxillofacial Surgery in Dogs and Cats* (1st edn), Saunders–Elsevier, Edinburgh, UK.

157 Illustrations reprinted with permission from Verstraete FJM, Van Aarde RJ, Nieuwoudt BA, Mauer E, Kas PH (1996). The dental pathology of feral cats on Marion Island. Part I: congenital, developmental and traumatic abnormalities. *Journal of Comparative Pathology,* **115**:265–82.

203 Illustration reproduced with permission from Tsugawa AJ, Lommer MJ, Verstraete FJM (2012). Extraction of canine teeth in dogs. In FJM Verstraete and MJ Lommer (eds) *Oral and Maxillofacial Surgery in Dogs and Cats* (1st edn), Saunders–Elsevier, Edinburgh, UK.

Suggested reading material

Anatomy
Constantinescu GM, Schaller O. *Illustrated Veterinary Anatomical Nomenclature.* 3rd ed. Stuttgart: Enke Verlag, 2011.
Evans HE, de Lahunta A. *Miller's Anatomy of the Dog.* 4th ed. Philadelphia: Elsevier Saunders, 2013.
Nanci A. *Ten Cate's Oral Histology: Development, Structure, and Function.* 8th ed. St. Louis: Elsevier Mosby, 2013.

Anesthesia
Tranquilli WJ, *et al.* (eds). *Lumb & Jones Veterinary Anesthesia and Analgesia.* 4th ed. Baltimore: Williams & Wilkins, 2007.

Dental materials
Anusavice KJ. *Philips' Science of Dental Materials.* 12th ed. Philadelphia: Elsevier Saunders, 2012.

Endodontics
Hargreaves KM, Berman LH. *Cohen's Pathways of the Pulp.* 11th ed. St. Louis: Elsevier Mosby, 2015.

Equine dentistry
Easley J, Dixon PM, Schumacher J. *Equine Dentistry.* 3rd ed. Philadelphia: Elsevier Saunders, 2010.

Exotic dentistry
Capello V, Gracis M, Lennox A. *Rabbit and Rodent Dentistry.* Lake Worth: Zoological Education Network, 2005.

Orthodontics
Proffit WR, Fields HW, Sarbar D. *Contemporary Orthodontics.* 5th ed. St. Louis: Elsevier Mosby, 2012.

Pathology
Regezi JA, Sciubba JJ, Jordan RCK. *Oral Pathology: Clinical Pathologic Correlations.* 6th ed. Philadelphia: Elsevier Saunders, 2011.

Periodontology
Newman MG, Takei H, Klokkevold PR, Carranza FA. *Carranza's Clinical Periodontology.* 12th ed. Philadelphia: Elsevier Saunders, 2014.

Wolf HF, Rateitschak KH, Rateitschak EM, Hassell TM. *Color Atlas of Dental Medicine – Periodontology*. 3rd ed. New York: Thieme Medical Publishers, 2005.

Radiology
DuPont GA, DeBowes LJ. *Atlas of Dental Radiography in Dogs and Cats*. St. Louis: Elsevier Saunders, 2009.
White SC, Pharoah MJ. *Oral Radiology: Principles and Interpretation*. 7th ed. St. Louis: Elsevier Mosby, 2013.

Restorative dentistry/prosthodontics
Heymann HO, Swift EJ, Ritter AV. *Sturdevant's Art and Science of Operative Dentistry*. 6th ed. St. Louis: Elsevier Mosby, 2012.
Shillingburg HT, Jacobi R, Brackett SE. *Fundamentals of Tooth Preparations for Cast Metal and Porcelain Restorations*. Chicago: Quintessence Publishing Co., 1987.

Small animal dentistry
Holmstrom SE, Frost P, Eisner ER. *Veterinary Dental Techniques*. 3rd ed. Philadelphia: WB Saunders, 2004.
Tutt C, Deeprose J, Crossley DA (eds). *BSAVA Manual of Small Animal Dentistry*. 3rd ed. Quedgeley: British Small Animal Veterinary Association, 2007.

Surgery
Verstraete FJM, Lommer MJ. *Oral and Maxillofacial Surgery in Dogs and Cats*. Edinburgh: Elsevier Saunders, 2012.

Classification of questions

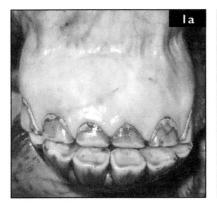
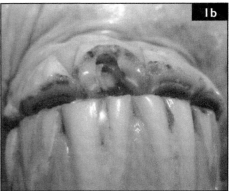

Question 1 During the examination of two horses (**1a, b**) on behalf of a prospective purchaser, an oral inspection was performed to assess age and oral conformation. What significance should be attached to the pattern of wear found on the incisor teeth?

Question 2 Compare in table form the reproduction of detail, dimensional stability, tear strength, maximum time until pouring, and comparative cost of alginate, reversible hydrocolloid, polyether, and vinyl polysiloxane impression materials.

Question 3 A wide variety of suture materials have been recommended for use in the oral cavity (**3a**).

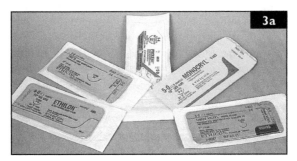

1 Chromic catgut persists in the human oral cavity for 4–7 days, which is considered to be ideal since this approximates the time limit for removal of non-absorbable suture material. Which synthetic suture material combines a rapid and predictable absorption time with minimal inflammatory response and minimal tissue drag?
2 What type of needle is recommended for intraoral suturing?

I–3: Answers

Answer 1 The pattern of wear on the maxillary incisor teeth arose by abrasion and is highly suggestive that the horses are crib-biters and/or wind-suckers. In many countries it is the legal responsibility of a vendor to declare whether or not a horse is free from stable vices (stereotypic behavior). However, in the face of the findings shown, the examining veterinarian should observe the resting horse carefully for any tendency to display these stereotypes, and in any event the client should be advised of the possible significance of the dental changes. Horses with this behavior can have endodontic disease from the abrasion and complicated fractures of the incisor crowns (**1b**).

Answer 2

	Alginate	Reversible hydrocolloid	Polyether	Vinyl polysiloxane
Reproduction of detail	Poor	Fair	Excellent	Excellent
Dimensional stability	Poor	Fair	Very good	Excellent
Tear strength	Very low	Very low	Moderate	High
Maximum time for pouring	Immediate	7 hours	7 days	14 days
Comparative cost	Very low	Low	Very high	High to very high

(See also **13** on the classification of impression materials)

Answer 3
1 Poliglecaprone 25 (Monocryl™, Ethicon, Inc., Somerville, NJ) (**3b**) is a synthetic, monofilament suture material that combines the rapid absorption comparable with that of catgut with the inertness, strength, and smoothness previously only found in monofilament, synthetic, non-absorbable suture materials such as polypropylene.
2 Although taper needles have been recommended in the past, small, swaged-on, 3/8-circle, reverse-cutting needles (e.g. FS-2 or P-3, Ethicon, Inc.) cause less tissue drag and are therefore recommended for intraoral suturing.

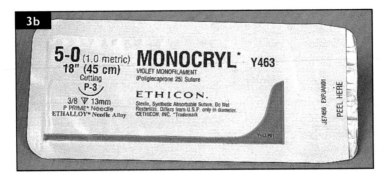

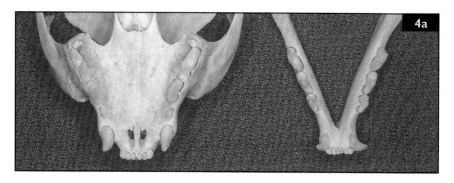

Question 4 The dental formula of the primitive mammalian consists of 44 teeth (3 incisor, 1 canine, 4 premolar, and 3 molar teeth in each quadrant). The modern carnivore dentition shows several adaptations of the primitive mammalian dentition.

1 Which teeth in the cat (**4a**) are reduced in number compared with the primitive mammalian dentition?
2 What is a carnassial tooth?
3 Which are the carnassial teeth in the cat?

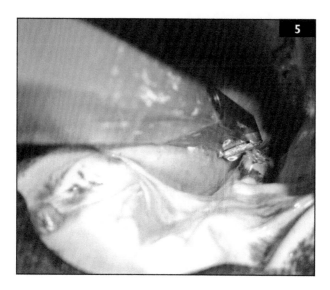

Question 5 What dental procedure is being performed in this photograph (**5**) and why?

4, 5: Answers

Answer 4
1 The premolar and molar teeth (**4b**). The maxillary first premolar tooth and mandibular first and second premolar teeth have disappeared in the modern cat dentition. The correct anatomic designations of the first premolar teeth actually seen in the upper and lower jaws are the maxillary second premolar tooth and mandibular third premolar tooth, respectively. Moreover, the cat only has one molar tooth per quadrant. This is the first molar tooth. The maxillary molar tooth is a small, non-functional, single- or double-rooted tooth and the mandibular molar tooth has lost its grinding surface and become a carnassial tooth.
2 A '*dens sectorius*'. The premolar teeth and especially the carnassial teeth are secodont, i.e. they have sharp cutting edges which function as scissors during jaw movement.
3 The maxillary fourth premolar and the mandibular first molar teeth.

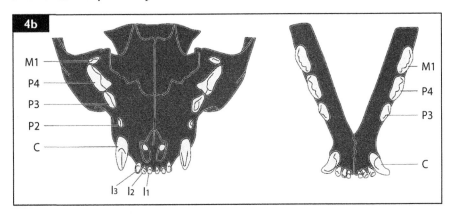

Answer 5 This is a motorized equine dental float used for occlusal adjustment. This entails removing the sharp enamel points from the buccal aspect of the maxillary cheek teeth and the lingual aspect of the mandibular cheek teeth. A float is also used to correct abnormalities such as tall or overlong teeth, hooks, ramps, and beaks, and to contour the mesial aspect of the second premolar teeth. Instrumentation utilized should allow the operator to perform precise corrections of the dental quadrants and cause minimal to no soft-tissue trauma.

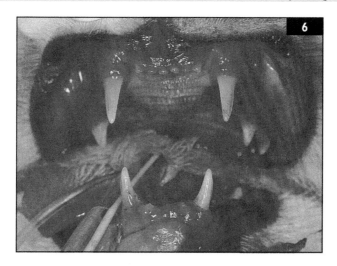

Question 6 This young adult cat is healthy with the exception of the oral disease shown (6) which is painful and results in anorexia. What would you recommend for medical management of this patient's oral problem?

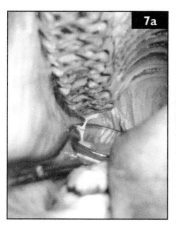

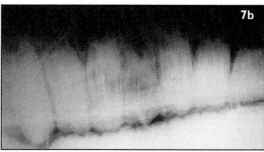

Question 7 A 12-year-old warmblood gelding was presented for a fetid nasal discharge from the left nostril and purulent discharge in the oral cavity (7a). What is the radiologic interpretation of the radiograph and treatment (7b)?

6, 7: Answers

Answer 6 This patient has severe gingivitis and stomatitis. Initial management of the acute, treatment-naïve patient would include a complete evaluation of the oral cavity and teeth, including full-mouth radiographs, complete periodontal treatment, and extraction of any teeth found to have resorption or significant periodontal bone loss. More often than not, diagnosis of this condition is delayed, and many stomatitis patients have significant secondary pathology related to the long-standing inflammation; often necessitating partial- to full-mouth extractions to address both the severe periodontitis that is present and also as a method of reducing the inflammation-eliciting, plaque-retentive surfaces of the tooth crowns (see 55). If neoplasia or other oral disease is suspected, a biopsy should be obtained for histopathology. Medical management of oral inflammatory disease is aimed at pain management and suppression of the inflammatory/immune response. Antibiotics may initially result in a partial improvement of the oral inflammation. Methylprednisolone (15–20 mg per cat, subcutaneously) generally results in significant improvement of oral inflammation, pain, and appetite. The duration of response depends on the severity of the oral inflammation; treatments generally are required every 3–6 weeks. Oral glucocorticoids (e.g. prednisolone) are usually not successful in initial management of severe inflammatory disease because of the inability to medicate; they may be used for long-term management in some cats with milder inflammation. Some cats show a better response to combination therapy with antibiotics and glucocorticoids. Long-term usage of corticosteroids may lead to insulin-resistant diabetes and is contraindicated in the presence of heart disease. Cyclosporine and feline omega interferon (Virbagen® Omega, Virbac) have been reported to be successful in the management of some cats with oral inflammatory disease; however, treatment in immunosuppressed cats should be carefully monitored.

Answer 7 The horse has a supernumerary left maxillary molar tooth. The tooth is sharing an alveolus with the left maxillary third molar tooth and subsequently there is no interproximal bone or periodontal ligament. There is a malocclusion due to the supernumerary tooth lacking opposing dentition. The impaction of food between the supernumerary tooth and the left maxillary third molar tooth has caused a periodontal-endodontic lesion with sinus involvement. There is also a radiolucent area in the reserve crown of the left maxillary first molar tooth seen orally as stage 2 infundibular caries that had been restored with composite.

Treatment in cases with supernumerary teeth, provided secondary conditions are not evident, includes frequent occlusal adjustments and imaging of the other dental quadrants for evidence of supernumerary teeth. Treatment in this case required extraction of the left maxillary third molar tooth and the supernumerary tooth with trephination and lavage of the left sinus compartments.

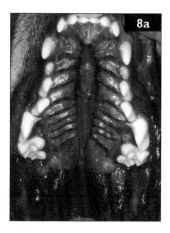

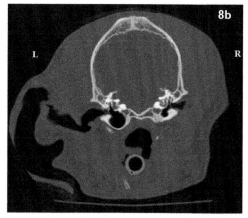

Question 8 Knowledge of palatal development helps in understanding facial malformations (**8a**).
1 What is the sequence of events in palatal development?
2 What other craniomaxillofacial abnormalities may be seen in conjunction with cleft lip and palate (**8b**)?

Question 9 The temporomandibular joint (TMJ) (**9**) is a condylar joint but it functions mainly like a hinge joint in carnivores.
1 Describe the anatomy of the TMJ.
2 What types of movement are possible?
3 What is the most common cause of TMJ pathology in the cat? Name two common conditions.
4 What is the most common type of TMJ luxation? Outline the management of such a case.

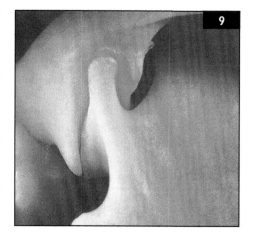

Answer 8

1 During embryogenesis, at about day 23, the paired maxillary processes, the paired mandibular processes and the median frontonasal process surround the primitive oral cavity (stomodeum). Median and lateral nasal processes originating from the frontonasal process extend on each side of olfactory placodes. In contrast to humans – where the upper lip is formed by the maxillary and nasal processes – in dogs and cats the upper lip and the primary palate are both formed by the midline fusion of the maxillary processes. At this stage of the development, the choanae open at the caudal end of the primary palate. Later, lateral palatine processes move towards the midline and fuse around day 33 with the nasal septum originating from the nasal process. This constitutes the secondary palate which will ossify (hard palate), except in the caudal part where it will form the soft palate. The genetic and non-genetic causes of cleft lip and palate have not been well documented in the dog and cat.

2 In a recent study, hypoplastic tympanic bullae (8b) were most commonly found in dogs with cleft lip and palate. Abnormalities can also be present in the nasal turbinates, nasal septum, vomer, and cribriform plate, frontal sinuses, and lateral ventricles.

Answer 9

1 The joint is comprised of the mandibular head of the condylar process of the mandible and the mandibular fossa of the temporal bone. An articular disk separates the joint into a dorsal and a ventral compartment. The disk is a flat fibrocartilaginous plate. The joint capsule is enforced by fibrous tissue which forms a strong ligament laterally. The caudoventral end of the zygomatic arch forms the retroarticular process which protects the joint and largely prevents caudal luxation.

2 The shapes of the condylar process of the mandible and the mandibular fossa of the temporal bone do not match exactly, which allows for some sliding movement as well as the hinge action. The sliding movements are very limited due to the precise interdigitation of teeth in the cat.

3 TMJ pathology in the cat usually occurs as a result of trauma. Two common conditions are luxation and fracture (intra-articular or periarticular).

4 Luxation is usually in a rostrodorsal direction. This causes rostromedial displacement of the mandible on the affected side and prevents closure of the mouth because of the resulting abnormal interlock of the teeth. Treatment of acute luxation consists of closing the animal's mouth with a wooden or plastic rod inserted between the maxillary fourth premolar teeth and mandibular first molar teeth and closing the mouth, pushing the mandible backwards until the head of the condylar process slips back into the mandibular fossa. Chronic luxation is best treated by condylectomy. Caudal luxation is less common, and may be associated with a fracture of the retroarticular process.

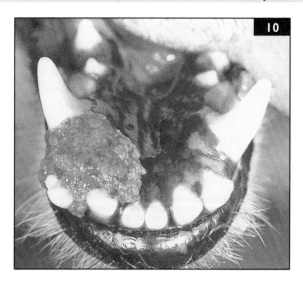

Question 10 There is continuing confusion with regard to the origin and nomenclature of 'epulides' in the dog (10). In broad terms, what is the current understanding and classification of these lesions and what is their clinical significance?

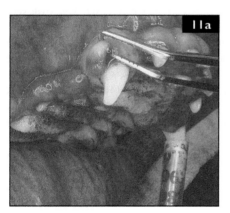
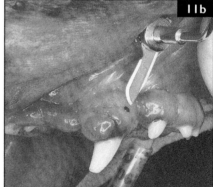

Question 11
1 What procedure is being performed here (11a, b)?
2 Discuss the principles, indications, and contraindications of this procedure.

Answer 10 The term *epulis* refers to any tumor or tumor-like lesion on the gingiva (10). It is a clinically descriptive term with no specific histopathologic connotation. Most authors agree that epulides can be classified into four groups: (1) A group of non-neoplastic, reactive lesions occurring as a result of chronic low-grade irritation, e.g. focal fibrous gingival hyperplasia and pyogenic granuloma. (2) Benign neoplastic lesions of odontogenic origin, e.g. peripheral odontogenic fibroma. (3) Canine acanthomatous ameloblastoma, previously known as the acanthomatous epulis, which is an infiltrating epithelial tumor. (4) Various malignant non-odontogenic tumor types, e.g. squamous cell carcinoma and fibrosarcoma.

The clinical importance of epulides can be summarized as follows: (1) An epulis must be biopsied. (2) If multiple lesions are present in an oral cavity, all must be biopsied. (3) Surgical margins for definitive excision must be determined by the biopsy result. (4) Appropriate dental treatment is indicated for reactive lesions.

Answer 11
1 Gingivectomy/gingivoplasty.
2 Gingivectomy is an excisional procedure performed to remove the diseased soft-tissue wall of a suprabony periodontal pocket or to remove gingival enlargement. Gingivoplasty signifies reshaping of the remaining gingival contour. The procedure is initiated by marking pocket depths with bleeding points on the surface of the mucosa. An incision is begun apical to the bleeding point to contour the gingiva physiologically and completely remove the pocket wall (**11c**). These bleeding points can be made with a probe or Goldman–Fox periodontal pocket-marking forceps (**11a**). Gingivectomy may be performed with gingivectomy knives (**11b**), cold steel blades, electrosurgery, laser, and dental burs. After excision, periodon-

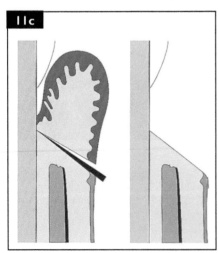

tal débridement is performed. Healing occurs after epithelial migration over the wound which takes 1 day for each 0.5–1 mm covered. For this reason, the gingivectomy bevel is not made greater than necessary to achieve good post-healing tissue contour.

Gingivectomy is indicated for gingival enlargement and associated pseudopockets. It is contraindicated in infrabony defects where incomplete pocket removal and reverse architecture would result. Also, a narrow and/or thin band of attached gingiva may preclude gingivectomy which might remove too much tissue.

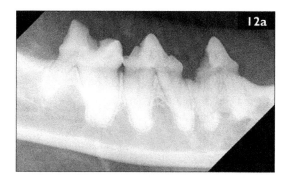

Question 12 Tooth resorption is one of the most common indications for tooth extraction.
1 Outline the challenges associated with extraction of teeth affected by resorption.
2 What are the American Veterinary Dental College types of resorption?
3 Describe the radiographic type of tooth resorption affecting these teeth (12a).
4 What is the recommended extraction technique?

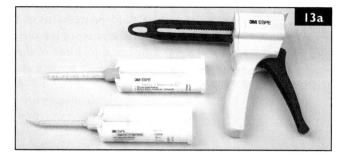

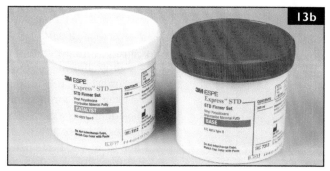

Question 13 How are impression materials classified (13a, b)? Give a concise, systematic classification of the various materials.

11

Answer 12

1 Perhaps the biggest challenge encountered when extracting teeth with tooth resorption is fracturing of the root, crown, or crown from the root. Not only are teeth with tooth resorption inherently structurally more brittle, depending on the radiographic type of the tooth resorption lesion, significant dentoalveolar ankylosis may be present, increasing the chance of iatrogenic tooth fracture during extraction.

2 (12b) Type 1. Normal root radiopacity; normal appearance of the periodontal ligament space; commonly identified in the cervical portion of the root and at the level of the furcation; often accompanied by alveolar bone loss.

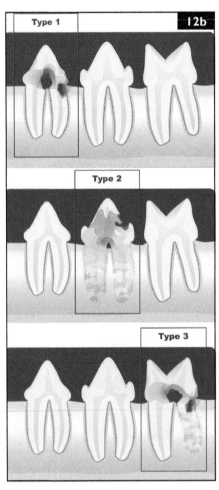

Type 2. Root density approximating the radiopacity of the alveolar bone; loss of the normal periodontal ligament space.

Type 3. Radiographic features of both type 1 and type 2.

3 Type 2 tooth resorption of the left mandibular third premolar tooth. Notice that the root density of the left mandibular third premolar tooth approximates the radiopacity of the surrounding alveolar bone, and loss of the normal periodontal ligament space architecture.

4 Although standard open surgical exodontic techniques are typically adequate for the extraction of resorbed teeth, intentional coronectomy may be a suitable treatment alternative for resorbed teeth with dentoalveolar ankylosis (type 2). Making the determination of whether intentional coronectomy is an appropriate option for treatment is tightly linked to the radiographic appearance of the lesion, and simply reverting to a coronectomy unless specific conditions exist (i.e. dentoalveolar ankylosis) is not appropriate, especially when there are severe periodontal pockets, stomatitis, immunocompromise, or

radiographically identifiable endodontic disease. Reasonable efforts should be extended to extract all type 1 and amenable portions of type 3 resorbed teeth. Radiographic typing prior to treating resorbed teeth is mandatory, as it will not only reduce the frustration level of the veterinarian, but will avoid unnecessary collateral trauma to the surrounding bone incurred during unsuccessful attempts at the retrieval of severely ankylosed roots. When performing an intentional coronectomy, the client should be notified of this decision, and the procedure should be appropriately noted in the dental record.

When performing an intentional coronectomy, the first step entails development of a full-thickness gingival envelope flap; which is followed by the actual coronectomy that is performed with a #701 carbide bur or other appropriate cutting bur on a high-speed or electric handpiece. A round diamond bur is then used to perform the alveoloplasty of the sharp buccal and lingual/palatal edges of the alveolar margin. It is also important to reduce the height of the alveolar bone after the coronectomy to facilitate closure of the flap. Closure is perhaps the most difficult aspect of the coronectomy procedure, which is intended as a conservative procedure, but actually requires conversion of the most conservative of flaps (envelope) beyond the mucogingival junction into the alveolar mucosa to provide a tension-free closure – this is especially challenging when closing canine and mandibular premolar–molar coronectomy sites. Proper flap development with adequate exposure also avoids trauma to the flap that may occur during use of the bur. The flap for the coronectomy site is sutured closed using an absorbable synthetic monofilament of the operator's choice in a simple interrupted pattern. Post-coronectomy radiographs should be obtained to ensure smoothness of the remaining alveolar margin, and that all recognizable crown and root have been removed.

Answer 13 There are two ways by which impression materials can be classified. One way to classify them is by setting process, which includes materials that harden by chemical reaction (irreversible) or are temperature-induced (reversible). Materials may also be classified by elasticity: whether the resulting product is elastic or inelastic. Inelastic materials are used for obtaining impressions from edentulous human patients, and are rarely used in veterinary dentistry, except for bite registration (i.e. waxes).

	Rigid (inelastic)	Elastic
Set by chemical reaction (irreversible)	Plaster	Irreversible hydrocolloids (alginates)
	Zinc oxide	Non-aqueous elastomers
Set by temperature change (reversible)	Wax	Reversible hydrocolloids

12, 13: Answers

The elastic impression materials include the irreversible hydrocolloids, better known as the alginates, which are commonly used in veterinary dentistry when obtaining impressions for study models. The reversible hydrocolloids are commonly referred to as hydrocolloids. They are rarely used in clinical human and veterinary dentistry, because of their poor flow and tear resistance, and because better modern impression materials are readily available, but are still widely used in the laboratory setting for the purposes of cast duplication. The non-aqueous elastomers are rubber-like materials. They are further classified according to chemistry (see chart below), but may also be classified by viscosity (heavy body or putty; regular body or medium viscosity, and light body, low viscosity or 'wash').

Types of non-aqueous elastomers	Comments
Polyether	e.g. Impregum™ (3M ESPE)
Polysulfide	e.g. COE-FLEX® (GC America)
Condensation polymerizing silicone	Replaced by the addition polymerizing silicones
Addition polymerizing silicone	Better known as vinyl polysiloxane, e.g. Imprint™ 4 (3M ESPE)

Vinyl polysiloxanes are the most commonly used impression materials in veterinary dentistry for the purposes of obtaining high-detail impressions for prosthetic crowns. Polyether impression materials, such as Impregum™ (3M ESPE), are also still available and are an excellent choice for high accuracy impressions under moist conditions due to their hydrophilicity. Both the polysulfides and condensation polymerizing silicones are mentioned here for completeness, but have largely been replaced by the aforementioned materials. COE-FLEX® (GC America), a polysulfide, is still available, but has very undesirable characteristics, including a slow set time, offensive odor, and high shrinkage once the water in the setting reaction has evaporated (i.e. models must be poured within 30–60 minutes).

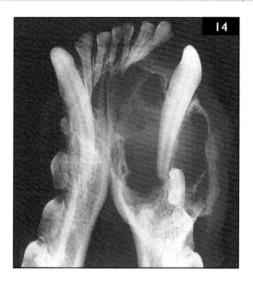

Question 14
1 How would you describe the radiologic findings associated with the oral mass found in this 3-year-old dog (14), and what is your tentative radiologic diagnosis?
2 Provided the radiologic diagnosis is confirmed on biopsy, what would be the recommended treatment and prognosis?

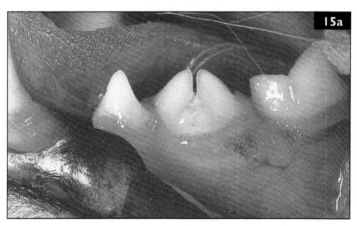

Question 15
1 What developmental disturbance in tooth shape is shown (15a)?
2 What other teeth in the dog and cat can be affected?
3 What are the related conditions?

Answer 14

1 This is a large, space-occupying lesion of the rostral part of the left mandible, expanding over the symphysis into the right mandible. The border of the lesion consists of thinned cortical bone, with little or no periosteal reaction. The overall radiographic density of the lesion is low and it seems to consist of one large cystic area with a few smaller ones on the periphery. The surrounding bone is expanded but the cortical bone is not disrupted. The left mandibular first premolar tooth is absent. The left mandibular canine tooth is marginally displaced but is no longer supported by bone. All left mandibular incisor teeth and to a lesser extent the right first and second incisor teeth are displaced. The tentative diagnosis is an intraosseous, benign tumor suggestive of a central (or intraosseous) ameloblastoma. This diagnosis was confirmed on biopsy.

2 A bilateral partial-rostral mandibulectomy would be indicated and would likely be curative. Adequate surgical margins would probably be mesial to the mandibular first molar tooth on the left and mesial to the third premolar tooth on the right. Metastasis of ameloblastoma in the dog has not been reported. A bilateral partial-rostral mandibulectomy that far distally is likely to result in the tongue hanging out and may necessitate tying off or repositioning the openings of the mandibular and sublingual salivary ducts.

Answer 15

1 This is a case of gemination of the mandibular fourth premolar tooth in a cat. Gemination is defined as an attempt to make two teeth from a single tooth germ, resulting in partial cleavage. A geminated single-rooted tooth usually has two incompletely separated crowns and a single root canal. In this case of a premolar tooth, three roots were present, the central one having a very wide root canal.

2 Gemination of single incisor teeth (15b) is relatively common in the dog, while geminated canine and premolar teeth in the dog and cat are rare. No reference to the occurrence of geminated molar teeth could be found. Gemination can also be present in the deciduous dentition.

3 Fusion and concrescence are related conditions. In cases of fusion, two tooth buds are united and the dentin is confluent. In cases of concrescence, the teeth are united by cementum only. If fusion occurs between two normal teeth, the total

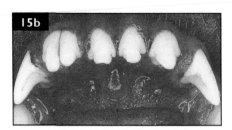

15b

number of teeth is reduced, which is not the case in gemination. However, it may not be possible to differentiate fusion of a normal tooth and an adjacent supernumerary tooth from a true geminated tooth. Twinning may be used to designate the presence of a normal and a supernumerary tooth of the same shape that are completely separate.

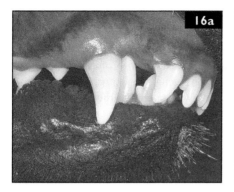
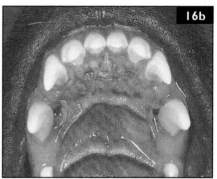

Question 16 The normal canine tooth occlusion in the dog comprises interdigitation of the mandibular canine teeth which diverge laterally, slotting evenly into the maxillary third incisor–canine interdental space without tooth-to-tooth contact. Palatal contact by malpositioned mandibular canine teeth is a commonly recognized malocclusion in domestic dogs (**16a, b**). Describe four different patterns of mandibular canine tooth malocclusion which commonly result in palatal trauma.

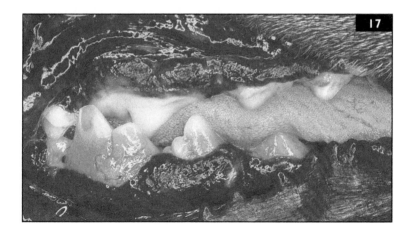

Question 17
1 What are the possible etiologies of the condition shown (**17**)?
2 Is there any functional impairment associated with this malocclusion?
3 Is any treatment indicated?

Answer 16 The four most common patterns of malocclusion resulting in palatal contact by the mandibular canine teeth are: (1) Lingual deviation of the mandibular canine teeth (upright canine teeth) in a normal-width jaw. This condition may be unilateral or bilateral. Under normal circumstances the mandibular canine teeth initially erupt in a rostrodorsal direction, using the pathway provided by the resorbing deciduous tooth root. Once the crown appears in the mouth, the tooth then tips laterally, so avoiding palatal contact. Sometimes the adult tooth erupts at an abnormal angle, leading directly to abnormal positioning. On other occasions, for whatever reason, the deciduous tooth root may not be resorbed, so that the permanent tooth is prevented from tipping laterally as it erupts. (2) An abnormally narrow ('base-narrow') mandible can result in the mandibular canine teeth contacting the palate even if they do diverge laterally at a normal angle. In many dogs with base-narrow mandibles the condition is masked by excessive lateral tipping of the canine teeth so that they do not cause palatal trauma. (3) Mandibular brachygnathism can lead to palatal injury by the mandibular canine teeth. In some cases the mandibular canine teeth are positioned level with the maxillary canine teeth which prevents the mandibular teeth tipping laterally. In more extreme cases there is a relative base-narrow effect due to the natural divergence of the maxillary dental arch distally. This is the case with an underdeveloped mandible (mandibular micrognathia), which is a skeletal malocclusion characterized by a mandible that is too narrow and too short. (4) A skeletal asymmetrical malocclusion, also referred to as 'wry mouth', may also result in palatal contact by one of the mandibular canine teeth.

Answer 17
1 A genetically narrow caudal maxilla or an abnormally wide mandible can result in a caudal crossbite. Trauma to the maxilla of a neonate or juvenile can result in a unilateral caudal crossbite.
2 There is generally no functional impairment resulting from caudal crossbite, except for possible abnormal attrition of premolar and/or molar teeth that are in occlusal contact.
3 Treatment is generally not indicated and would technically be very difficult.

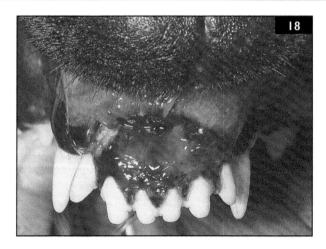

Question 18 This is an intraoral view of the rostral maxilla area of a 7-month-old intact female Labrador retriever, which was kicked in the mouth by a horse (**18**). Palpation and intraoral radiographic evaluation revealed a segmental fracture of the incisive bones involving an interdental bone fracture between the left maxillary second and third incisor teeth and the right maxillary second and third incisor teeth. The fracture segment contained the left and right maxillary first and second incisor teeth.

1 What is your diagnosis and treatment of the soft-tissue injury?
2 What non-invasive, inexpensive technique could be utilized to stabilize the segmental fracture of the rostral maxillary region?
3 What postoperative dental complications may be associated with this type of injury?

Question 19 A 16-month-old gelding has sustained trauma to the left maxillary incisor quadrant with buccal luxation of the left maxillary first and second incisor teeth (**19a**). What is a simple yet effective method to restore normal occlusal alignment and to provide stability of the teeth during healing?

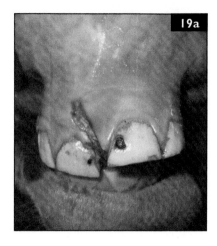

Answer 18

1 This is a midline avulsion of the gingiva from the maxilla. Initial therapy in these cases should include thorough débridement and flushing of the wound. Following thorough débridement, the avulsed gingiva is sutured to the palatal mucosa with fine, monofilament, absorbable suture material. Sutures may be placed around adjacent teeth to improve the retention of sutures.

2 The incisive fracture segment contains the right and left maxillary first and second incisor teeth. The maxillary second and third incisor teeth are interdentally wired to each other on the left and right to provide initial reduction of the fracture site. Once the fracture segment is reduced, an intraoral composite splint is applied to the facial aspect and the interdental spaces of the six maxillary incisor teeth to provide semi-rigid stabilization until fracture healing occurs.

3 The trauma sustained to the incisive bones may result in postoperative endodontic disease of the maxillary incisor teeth. Although the incisor teeth were not fractured in this case, periodontal trauma (concussion, subluxation) can displace the root apex and compromise the blood supply to the pulp. Pulp that is impaired or devoid of a blood supply may become colonized by bacteria via hematogenous spread through the apical foramen, resulting in pulpitis or pulp necrosis. Periodic re-evaluation of the rostral maxilla region will determine the need for subsequent endodontic therapy in this case.

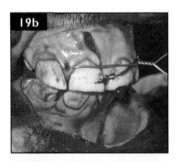

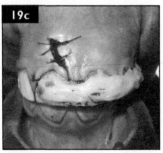

Answer 19 Radiographs are obtained to determine the extent of the trauma. Teeth with root fractures or in cases where the teeth have lost nearly all periodontal attachment should have extraction considered. Simple in-and-out wire fixation with monofilament steel is very effective for the fixation of incisor quadrant fractures of the mandible or maxilla (**19b**). The canine teeth provide stabilizing points but when these are not present in mares, geldings, or young horses, a lag screw inserted at the buccal aspect at an equivalent level can be used. Normal occlusion is checked after removal of the endotracheal tube. Absorbable sutures are used to close the mucosal wounds (**19c**). Care should be taken to protect the soft tissues from laceration by the sharp ends of the fixation wire. This can be achieved either by tucking the ends between teeth or by covering them with a dental composite. In this case the left maxillary third incisor tooth was not affected and could be used as an anchor point. A small groove was made on the distal aspect of the tooth for the wire to set in.

Question 20 This dog was presented with an acute inability to close the mouth but no lateral deviation of the mandible (20).
1 What is your tentative clinical diagnosis?
2 How can this diagnosis be confirmed?
3 Presuming that the tentative diagnosis is confirmed, what is the treatment?

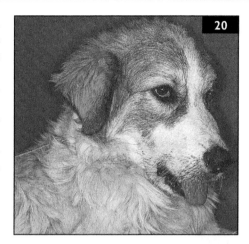

Question 21 An 8-year-old, neutered male cat was presented for evaluation of violent episodic left-sided mouth pawing, 'as if trying to remove something from the mouth,' with exaggerated licking and chewing movements that seemed to occur after eating or grooming. The client reported that the patient experienced similar symptoms as a kitten, but that the episodes were milder and resolved without treatment. Anesthetized oral and radiographic examination of the patient revealed tooth resorption lesions at both mandibular third premolar teeth, and unilateral self-mutilation injury to the tongue (21). The teeth with resorption lesions were extracted and an Elizabethan collar was applied to discourage and minimize the effects of the mutilation.

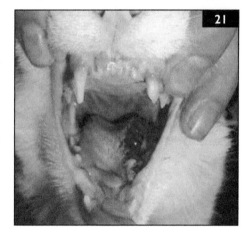

1 What condition is described in this cat?
2 What treatment is recommended for this condition?

Answer 20

1 Bilateral traumatic luxation of the temporomandibular joint.

2 The diagnosis is confirmed by radiography or preferably computed tomography. Two views are currently in use: the dorsoventral closed-mouth skull radiograph and the closed-mouth lateral oblique view (15–20°, nose tilted up). Unilateral or bilateral luxation is radiologically evidenced by the fact that the condylar process is not located within the mandibular fossa. Capsular osteophyte formation is evidence of a long-standing or recurrent luxation. Usually, the condylar process displaces rostrodorsally. If unilateral, the animal is presented with a typical lateral deviation to the side opposite the luxated joint.

3 Reduction is accomplished under general anesthesia by forcing the condyle ventrally. This can be done by inserting a fulcrum (e.g. pencil, syringe, dowel – depending on patient size) in between the molar teeth and gently forcing the mouth closed; this in turn levers the condylar process in a ventrocaudal direction back into the mandibular fossa. Aftercare may include the use of a tape muzzle. Recurrent and chronic luxations can be treated by condylectomy.

Answer 21

1 Feline orofacial pain syndrome (FOPS) is a poorly understood neuropathic disorder with a predominance in the Burmese cat that results in episodic, typically unilateral, signs of oral pain; often resulting in severe self-mutilation injury to the face and tongue. The condition appears to be triggered by mouth activity (e.g. eating, drinking, grooming) or environmental stress, and affected cats often (63%) have concurrent oral disease and dysfunction of sensory trigeminal nerve processing that causes paroxysmal firing of the trigeminal nerve. Any age cat can be affected with FOPS. Cats often exhibit initial symptoms as a kitten at the time of permanent tooth eruption, and the condition frequently recurs later in life. FOPS is a diagnosis of exclusion and all predisposing medical, dental, and behavioral problems should be ruled out before chronic treatment is instituted.

2 Management of FOPS should start with the treatment of existing dental disease, especially tooth resorption, which is a common associated condition, and followed by medical therapy. Medical therapeutic options include traditional analgesic medications (e.g. opioids, NSAIDs) for mild cases, and gabapentin with or without anti-epileptic drugs for longer-term control in the majority of cases. Anti-epileptics such as phenobarbital are believed to be effective for the treatment of FOPS due to their anti-allodynic effects and not for their anti-convulsant effects. Deterrents to mutilation such as Elizabethan collars, paw bandaging, and vinyl nail caps (Soft Paws®) should be immediately implemented to minimize injury while the primary cause of the pain is investigated and treated.

Question 22 This cat has a membranous bulge lingual to the mandibular first molar tooth (**22**).
1 Of what does this membranous bulge consist?
2 Is there an equivalent structure in the dog?
3 What consequences would you expect if this bulge was removed?

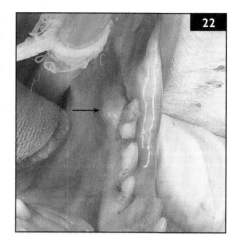

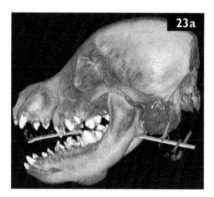

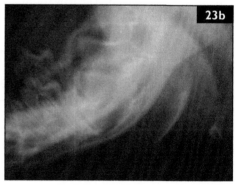

Question 23 A 5-month-old castrated male West Highland White terrier dog was presented for ptyalism, decreased interest in playing with toys, and anorexia. Examination revealed temporal muscle atrophy, and painful firm swellings of the left mandibular body and caudal to the right mandible. Opening of the jaws elicited discomfort, and was reduced, with a maximum interincisal measurement of 40 mm. The patient was also febrile at 104°F (40°C). A cone-beam CT of the skull was obtained (**23a**).
1 Describe the CT findings.
2 What is the diagnosis?
3 What is the recommended treatment?
4 What similar condition has been described in immature large-breed dogs (**23b**)?

Answer 22
1 A small, mixed-salivary gland.
2 No. The ferret, however, has a gland of similar location to the cat.
3 A specific function for this gland has not been reported. Following excisional biopsy of this structure, there were no clinical changes evident in tongue function, moistness of the mouth, or calculus deposition.

Answer 23
1 The three-dimensional reconstructed volume rendering of the skull (23a) of the dog shows a smooth hyperostosis of the left mandibular body at the level of the left mandibular fourth premolar and first molar teeth with an extensive bead-like osseous proliferation on the left tympanic bulla.
2 Craniomandibular osteopathy (CMO) is a non-neoplastic condition of the West Highland White terrier, Scottish terrier, Boston terrier, and Cairn terrier (and less commonly in 20 or more other non-terrier breeds), that results in painful, often bilateral, swellings of the bones of the skull – mandible, tympanic bullae and other bones of the cranium. The calvarium and tentorium ossium are also often thickened. In severe cases permanent restriction of the TMJ may occur, although in the majority of cases, the symptoms as well as the swellings resolve to nearly undetectable levels by the time of skeletal maturity at 11–13 months of age. A waxing and waning fever, as high as 104°F (40°C), 3–4 days' duration, may be seen during periods of bone proliferation every 2–4 weeks. Affected dogs are typically diagnosed between 4–7 months of age and dogs may be of either gender. The inheritance pattern of the trait of CMO is believed to be monogenic (controlled by a single gene), and inherited as a simple autosomal recessive trait. A CMO genetic test is available; responsible breeding practices have significantly decreased the prevalence of this disease since it was first reported in Britain nearly 60 years ago.
3 Non-steroidal anti-inflammatory drugs or anti-inflammatory-dose corticosteroids, and other analgesics are prescribed as needed until symptoms resolve. Symptoms will usually wax and wane in 10–14-day pain/fever cycles, so it is not unusual for CMO patients to feel better during these brief respites even without medications.
4 Periostitis ossificans (PO) is a swelling of the mandible that has been described in immature large-breed dogs (23b). PO is a self-resolving condition that has a characteristic radiographic appearance of a two-layered (double) ventral mandibular margin. Histopathology of the affected bone is consistent with periosteal new bone formation. Although the cause of PO is often unknown, it is believed to be the result of an undulating infection, a chronic active osteomyelitis that creates an 'onion-skinned' layering of the mandibular cortex when there is an alternating pattern of infection-related lifting of the periosteum followed by new bone formation.

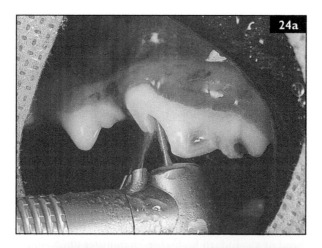

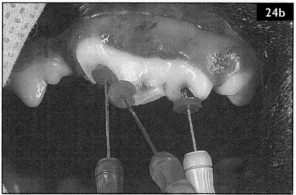

Question 24 These pictures show the transcoronal access to the roots of the maxillary fourth premolar tooth in a 6-year-old dog (**24a, b**). Describe why this approach is used.

Question 25 With regard to the transcoronal access in **24**:
1 Is making additional access sites preferable to accessing all three root canals via the fracture exposure site that is revealed when a large buccal slab fracture or central cusp fracture has exposed the pulp?
2 Is it important to preserve the palatal root when performing standard root canal therapy?

24, 25: Answers

Answer 24 The technique removes relatively little tooth substance so that maximum strength is preserved. The technique also provides straight-line access and good exposure to all three roots of the maxillary fourth premolar tooth, and can be performed in dogs of all sizes and breeds. The palatal root canal of the maxillary fourth premolar tooth is particularly difficult to thoroughly débride and shape for four reasons. First, this canal is often very small and, especially in older dogs, can be partially calcified. Second, the canal's exit from the pulp chamber is not in the same relative location in every tooth. Third, the palatal root varies in its relative orientation to the other roots. Sometimes it runs fairly parallel to the mesiobuccal root and sometimes it diverges from the mesiobuccal root. These last two factors make it difficult to locate the entrance to the canal from near the central cusp or from a site near the buccal groove. The fourth problem is encountered when trying to access the canal directly through the cusp of the palatal root. The cusp is small, and in many large dogs it is awkward or impossible to place the head of a standard high-speed handpiece close enough to drill a hole in the palatal cusp directly over the pulp chamber of this root. The transcoronal approach, which usually requires two new access sites, provides straight-line access to the apex of all three root canals being treated so that each canal can be adequately prepared.

Answer 25
1 Although it is often possible to access all three root canals through the fracture exposure site, complications are more prevalent due to increased pulp chamber perforations (over-instrumentation) of both the mesiobuccal and the palatal roots, metal fatigue leading to separated files if files are pre-bent, stripping the canal with the file's concave side and leaving contamination on the convex side of the prepared root canal, and the resultant ledging and filling voids (incomplete fills).
2 Yes. When palatal root canal complications occur, usually as a result of either over-instrumentation or inability to access the canal, clinicians may advocate amputating the palatal root to avoid subsequent periapical or periodontal disease. The palatal root, however, provides an important buttress effect against the powerful shearing forces exerted on the maxillary fourth premolar tooth and should be treated and preserved if at all possible. In a retrospective study, 20% of the maxillary fourth premolar teeth that had palatal roots amputated experienced crown fracture within 12 months of the procedure. Postoperatively, most dogs will continue to abuse this tooth by chewing on bones and other hard objects. With the transcoronal approach, fewer complications arise than with other techniques, and maximal strength and structure can be maintained in this large and important tooth.

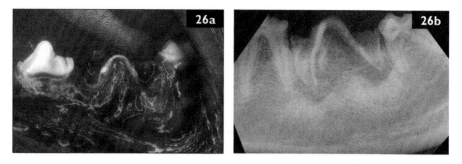

Question 26 An attempted simple extraction of this mandibular first molar tooth was not successful (**26a, b**). How can this complication be prevented?

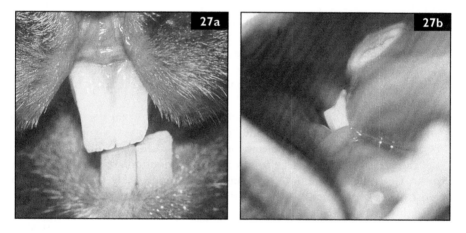

Question 27 This rabbit was approximately one year old. It had been fed on a concentrate ration (pellets and grain) without access to fresh herbage or hay since weaning.
1 What abnormality/abnormalities can be seen (**27a, b**)?
2 What is/are the likely cause(s)?
3 How significant is this in a 6-month-old rabbit compared with the same problem in an 8-year-old rabbit?

26, 27: Answers

Answer 26 This complication can be prevented by performing a surgical (open) rather than a simple (non-surgical or closed) extraction. This includes raising a gingival or mucogingival flap, a partial alveolectomy, and sectioning the tooth. Access to this area is frequently improved and the risk of soft-tissue injury reduced by raising a gingival or mucogingival flap. If necessary, a portion of the buccal alveolar bone can be removed to visualize the furcation and reduce root retention. It is easiest to ensure that a tooth is sectioned in the right place by starting cutting at the furcation. The instrument of choice to section multirooted teeth is a crosscut taper–fissure or coarse diamond taper bur in a high-speed dental handpiece. Each segment of the tooth should be treated as a single-rooted tooth. As much as possible of the periodontal ligament is severed using dental luxators or elevators. The rotational use of an elevator between tooth segments or on the alveolar margin bone aids extraction.

Answer 27
1 Oblique wear of the incisor teeth (**27a**). The mandible is also displaced to the left. As the abnormal wear pattern is slanting in the same direction it is likely that the mandibular position is significant, particularly as the rabbit was conscious when the photograph was taken. Rabbits have a normal wide range of lateral mandibular movement, so this positioning could have been caused by the method of restraint.
2 The abnormal wear pattern suggests a functional problem associated with lateral chewing movements. This could be due to skeletal, neurologic, muscular, or temporomandibular joint problems, or intraoral pathology. Abnormal wear of the cheek teeth (**27b**) can lead to physical restriction in the range of jaw movement. Conscious alteration of chewing pattern is probably the most common cause of subtle abnormalities such as this.

In this particular case, the diet was easily chewed, little grinding being required before the food was swallowed. When fed such a diet there is a tendency for rabbits to make reduced lateral chewing movements, resulting in insufficient wear to the lingual surfaces of the mandibular and buccal surfaces of the maxillary cheek teeth. In the case illustrated here the rabbit had developed sharp spikes only on the lingual surface of the mandibular cheek teeth on the right-hand side of its mouth. Occlusal adjustment to return the teeth to their normal contour, followed by introduction of a more abrasive (normal) diet of hay and fresh grass, which required considerable chewing effort, prevented recurrence over a 5-year follow-up period.
3 The significance of dental problems in animals with continuously growing teeth generally declines with age. If a minor abnormality has taken 8 years to develop it is not likely to progress rapidly, making successful long-term control much more likely. In a young animal such problems are frequently an indication that ongoing control measures will be required.

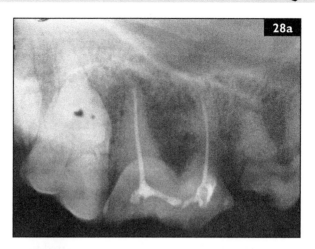

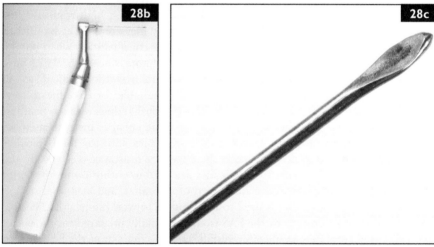

Question 28 Root canal therapy of teeth with long and narrow root canals, as seen on this radiograph (**28a**), can be difficult, but the key to success lies in the careful cleaning and shaping of the endodontic system. A number of techniques are available for cleaning and shaping. Explain the principles of the LightSpeed® technique (**28b, c**).

28: Answer

Answer 28 The steps of a routine standard root canal therapy include: (1) Access to the pulp chamber and root canal. (2) Pulpectomy or removal of the contents of the pulp chamber and the root canal. (3) Cleaning and shaping of the canal. (4) Obturation of the pulp cavity. (5) Restoration of the access opening(s).

LightSpeed® LSX™ files are non-tapered, stamped, nickel–titanium rotary files which have a non-cutting shaft and a short cutting blade. These files are available in an assortment of lengths – 21, 25, 31, and 50 mm. Dissimilar to traditional 0.04 taper files, LightSpeed® files avoid overpreparation of the middle third of the canal and underpreparation of the apical third of the file, safely avoiding common complications such as ledging, zipping and transportation.

The first step of instrumentation using the LightSpeed® LSX™ system is achieving straight-line access, followed by cleaning and shaping of the coronal one-third of the pulp cavity using traditional Gates–Glidden drills, or specialized coronal-tapering files with an unique 0.20 taper (LightSpeed® CRX™). Next, the working length is verified radiographically. Compared to the majority of rotary endodontic systems, the LightSpeed® technique requires a high rpm of 2,000–3,000 rpm; whereas the majority of tapered rotary files are used at significantly lower speeds of 300–600 rpm; this is an important consideration when purchasing an endodontic motor (and attachments). Also of note, since LSX™ files have a built-in safety mechanism where the file will separate from the handle if stressed, leaving a significant coronal length of the file available for easy file retrieval, the auto-torque reverse settings on the endodontic handpiece can typically be disabled. Once the working length is achieved, the canal is instrumented with smaller-sized to progressively larger-sized LSX™ files until the final apical size (FAS) is reached. The FAS is defined as the file where resistance is felt 4 mm short of working length. Sequentially larger files are used to within 6 mm of working length to clean and shape the middle third of the canal, and as a final step, the FAS file is reintroduced and is used to recapitulate to working length. The shape of the apical 4 mm created by the FAS is now optimally prepared for the use of a carrier-based gutta-percha plug (SimpliFill®) of the same size as the FAS. Alternatively, traditional cold gutta-percha cones can be cut to fit.

During the filing and shaping, flushing solutions (usually warm sodium hypochlorite) are used between each file change to flush debris and dentin filings from the canal. The tip of the endodontic flushing needle should reach within 1–2 mm of the apex, since effective flushing only occurs coronally to the needle tip. Also, the canal must be wide enough to prevent binding, since a lodged needle causes the canal to become an extension of the needle, resulting in direct tissue injection of the flushing solution into the periapical tissues. Alternatively, an apical negative-pressure rinsing-suctioning system specifically designed for endodontic use (EndoVac®) can be used.

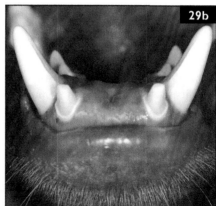

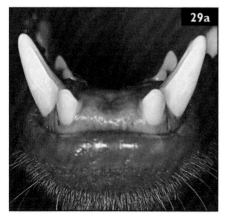

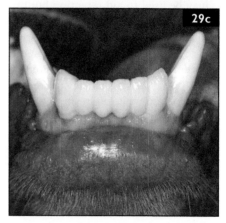

Question 29 This is an example of a ceramic bridge used for the replacement of four traumatically lost mandibular first and second incisor teeth in a dog (**29a–c**). How would you classify this type of bridge, and name its components?

Question 30 The photograph (**30**) shows a working dog with a maxillary fourth premolar tooth restored with a prosthetic crown. This crown has been in place for nearly 4 years.
1 What kind of material can be used for crown restoration in dogs?
2 Discuss the choice of alloy and the shape of such crowns.

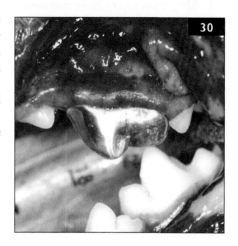

29, 30: Answers

Answer 29 A six-unit, fixed-fixed bridge: it is a one-piece bridge with the retainers fixed at either end of the pontics, consisting of six dental units. The portion of the bridge replacing the missing incisor teeth is known as the pontics. The pontics are suspended by two retainers, in this case jacket crowns, placed on the abutment teeth, the third incisor teeth. The connecting ceramic (known as joints) between the retainers and pontics may be stained to create the illusion of interdental spaces.

Answer 30
1 A prosthetic crown is an artificial restoration which replaces a part of the natural crown of the tooth. There are various types of crowns made of various materials. A crown can consist of a cap (jacket or full crowns) to protect the remaining crown substance, or it can be made as a combined post–crown prosthesis. A post may be used to aid retention but this weakens the root and increases the risk of subsequent root fracture. A tooth-colored crown can be made by fusing porcelain to a metal shell; however, the porcelain layer is fragile and this technique requires the removal of more dental substance. A recent development in the field of prosthodontics is the use of computer-aided design and computer-aided manufacturing (CAD/CAM) dentistry to create prosthetic crowns milled from solid blocks of ceramic or composite resin (see **130**).

Full-metal crowns are most commonly used and many different alloys are available. Non-precious alloys are silver-colored, inexpensive, and very hard; however, they are not cosmetic and are prone to black discoloration. Gold alloys are gold-colored, softer but esthetically more pleasing; pure gold is too soft for use as prosthetic crowns but many gold alloys are suitable for use in dogs. The biomechanical properties of the ideal alloy should meet but not exceed greatly those of the natural tooth.

2 Alloy crowns are most commonly used in veterinary dentistry. The composition of the alloy is normally chosen in consultation with the dental laboratory preparing the crown. The choice depends on strength, cost, and corrosion resistance. The metal crown should be made slightly shorter and with a rounder tip than the original tooth to minimize occlusal and shearing forces.

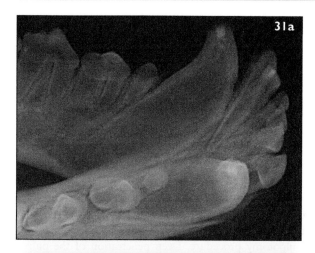

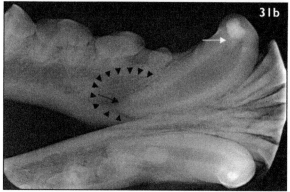

Question 31 A 7-month-old German Shepherd dog was presented for evaluation and treatment of a linguoverted right mandibular canine tooth that was traumatically occluding into the opposing hard palate mucosa. To address the traumatic malocclusion, the tooth was treated by crown-height reduction and vital pulp therapy using calcium hydroxide (also known as partial coronal pulpectomy and vital pulpotomy). Shown here are the postoperative radiograph (31a) and the 21-month follow-up radiograph (31b).

1 Describe the radiographic findings in the postoperative radiograph (31a) and follow-up radiograph (31b).
2 What is another protective dressing material that can be used for vital pulp therapy?
3 What parameters can be evaluated on radiographs to determine if the vital pulp therapy procedure has been successful?

31: Answer

Answer 31

1 The immediate post-treatment radiograph (**31a**) shows a wide pulp cavity and open apices of a right mandibular canine tooth consistent with the young age of the dog. Procedurally, a crown-height reduction and vital pulp therapy have been performed with deep penetration of the radiopaque pulp dressing material (calcium hydroxide) into the pulp chamber of the tooth. The 21-month follow-up radiograph (**31b**) shows a right mandibular canine tooth with tertiary dentin-bridge formation (white arrow), closed apices, and a comparatively narrow pulp cavity width and thicker dentin walls consistent with a tooth that survived post-treatment, but subsequently succumbed to pulp necrosis as evidenced by the well-defined periapical radiolucency (black arrowheads) and early external inflammatory root resorption (black arrow). Formation of a tertiary dentin bridge does not prevent pulp inflammation and necrosis through microleakage of bacteria through tubules and tunnels. The quality of the composite restoration and intermediate base are more crucial barriers to microleakage and success of the vital pulpotomy procedure. Deep penetration of the pulp dressing material into the vital pulp, rather than remaining as a distinct interface between the pulp and the restoration, is significantly associated with an increased risk of vital pulp therapy failure. Penetration of the dressing is more common in younger dogs with wider pulp cavities, and when an inadequate blood clot forms prior to application of the dressing.

2 Mineral trioxide aggregate (MTA) used as a pulp cavity dressing has superior biocompatibility compared to calcium hydroxide because it does not result in a necrotic cell layer between the dressing and the pulp. The quality of the tertiary dentin bridge that develops with MTA has also been shown to provide a tighter seal attributable to less porosity and resistance to dissolution compared to tertiary dentin bridges formed with calcium hydroxide. A recent study that evaluated the factors associated with the outcome of vital pulp therapy showed that MTA performed favorably as a pulp dressing material for vital pulp therapy with a 92% success rate compared to vital pulp therapies performed with calcium hydroxide which had a 58% success rate. Vital pulp therapy requires specialized equipment, materials, and skill to perform correctly, and is extremely technique sensitive, but when performed well, may achieve successful clinical results similar to standard root canal therapy, which has a 94% success rate.

3 One can compare the width of the pulp cavity with the pre-treatment radiographs, and see the continued secondary dentin deposition, and screen for periapical changes. Both occlusal and lateral radiographic views of the treated tooth and contralateral tooth should be obtained to increase the likelihood of detecting subtle periapical changes and differentiating true periapical disease from chevron artifacts. Radiographic follow-up may be performed as early as 3 months post-treatment, but should be obtained no later than 6 months following treatment, and annually thereafter. Although many early treatment failures will be detected between 12–23 months, longer-term follow-up is necessary to detect late failures. Tooth color and transillumination of the tooth are additional, but more subjective, methods to determine pulp vitality.

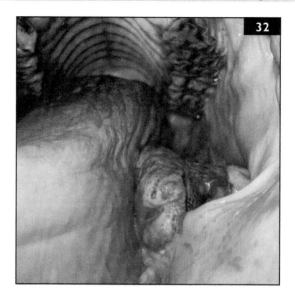

Question 32 What should be included in the diagnostic work-up of this horse's oral cavity (32)?

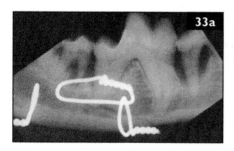
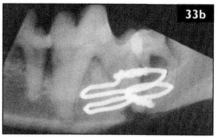

Question 33 These are two intraoral radiographs depicting the use of intraosseous wiring for the repair of a bilateral mandibular fracture in a dog (33a, b).
1 What is the most important principle in the management of jaw fractures? List several additional principles that should be utilized in the management of these fractures.
2 What is the proper technique for tightening wires during the fixation of jaw fractures?

32, 33: Answers

Answer 32 There is a large soft-tissue mass affecting the lingual and buccal surface of the left mandible. The teeth of the dental quadrant demonstrate the typical staining noted when the horse avoids mastication with the dental quadrants. Tannins in the feed material produce a brown staining that covers the occlusal surface.

Radiographs, and ideally computed tomography with tridimensional reconstruction, should be obtained to determine the extent of bone involvement. Incisional biopsy of the mass and lymph node aspirates are indicated.

Neoplastic processes in the oral cavity of the horse include squamous cell carcinoma, odontogenic tumors and other tumor types. Many have a poor prognosis and treatment options are limited, depending on the site of the tumor. This was a case of fibrosarcoma with invasion of the mandible and involvement of several premolar teeth.

Answer 33

1 Restoration of occlusion and anatomic reduction of the fracture. The interdigitation of the teeth is precise and the tolerance for error is narrow. Proper dental occlusion results from anatomic reduction of fracture fragments. However, proper occlusion may be difficult to achieve when there has been bone loss or loss of teeth, or when the fracture is highly comminuted. In these cases it is important to rely on occlusion of the remaining teeth as a guide and accept less-than-perfect bone reduction if necessary. In cases in which there has been bone loss or loss of teeth, an alternative technique for jaw fracture repair other than intraosseous wiring is recommended. Additional guidelines for the application of intraosseous wiring in the treatment of jaw fractures include the following: (1) A ventral surgical approach is recommended. (2) Tension band principles should be utilized. (3) Soft alveolar bone, reactive bone, or infected bone should be avoided during wire placement. (4) Wires should be placed somewhere between perpendicular to the fracture line and parallel to the long axis of the mandibular body, and if two wires are used, they should be placed at an angle to each other. (5) All orthopedic wires should be fastened securely. (6) Additional support should be utilized if necessary. (7) At least two wires should be placed across any single fracture line. (8) Excessive soft-tissue dissection and the incorporation of soft tissue beneath wires should be avoided.

In the case illustrated, complications can be expected because: (1) There are teeth present in the fracture lines. (2) The wires placed in the left mandible are parallel, allowing a swivel action. (3) Multiple fractures are present, exceeding the limits of what can reasonably be expected of intraosseous wiring.

2 Wires should be preplaced before tightening. While the wire is being tightened, tension should be applied to the wire to ensure that a tight fit of the wire is achieved. Proper wire tightening allows the wire to twist around itself rather than one wire twisting around the other. Following wire placement, occlusive alignment should be re-evaluated. This is easily achieved when the patient has been intubated via pharyngotomy (see **81**).

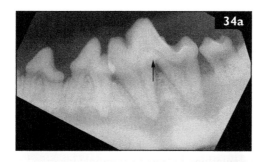

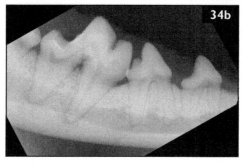

Question 34 A 3-year-old, neutered male Jack Russell terrier was presented for evaluation of a chronic fluctuant intermandibular swelling that had previously been treated by incision-drainage of purulent material and several courses of antibiotic therapy. Oral examination revealed a parulis and extraoral draining tract associated with the left mandibular first molar tooth. Upon closer inspection of the tooth a subtle indentation and discoloration of the enamel in the crown at the level of the furcation was identified. Intraoral dental radiographs (34a) revealed a smooth-margined widening of the ventral margin of the mandible apical to the left mandibular first molar tooth, severe horizontal bone loss with furcation exposure, vertical bone loss at the distal root that fuses with a periapical radiolucency at the same root (type 3 periodontal–endodontic lesion), radiopacity (arrowheads) in the furcation region of the crown, and well-defined periapical radiolucencies at both roots that exited through the ventral margin at the mesial root. Radiographs of the right mandibular first molar tooth (34b) revealed moderate horizontal bone loss with furcation involvement, ill-defined periapical radiolucencies at both roots, and a radiopacity (arrow) in furcation region of the crown.

1 What condition is described in this dog?
2 What treatment options should be considered for this condition?

Question 35 Cortical blindness in cats has been reported following anesthetized dental procedures. What is a proposed mechanism for this complication?

34, 35: Answers

Answer 34

1 This condition is referred to as dens invaginatus, or by its synonym (dens-in-dente), and is an uncommon developmental anomaly of permanent teeth, and less commonly deciduous teeth, where there is an infolding or invagination of the enamel into the dentin, periodontal ligament space, and in some cases directly into the pulp chamber. The enamel lining is often incomplete, creating portals of entry for bacteria and other irritants into the pulp and periodontal ligament space that may lead to pulp necrosis, periapical pathosis, and sometimes combined periodontal–endodontic disease. Dens invaginatus in the dog, as it is in humans, is often symmetrical in presentation; it is most commonly identified at the buccal aspect of the tooth in dogs, whereas in humans, lesions are typically present palatally.

2 Treatment options include prophylactic restoration of the area of infolding, standard (or surgical) root canal therapy, and extraction. In many cases, restoration of the invagination is not an option, since lesions are often identified late in the course of disease where periapical pathosis is already present, or treatment would be extremely challenging due to the proximity of the defect to the furcation. When restorative treatment is attempted, serial radiographic follow-up is required. Defects frequently extend subgingivally and contain numerous fine canals, necessitating flap development to achieve a dry working area and making closure of all portals difficult to impossible. Because of the propensity for teeth with this condition to lose vitality, performing endodontic therapy prior to restoration is not an unreasonable option.

Answer 35 Metal spring-loaded mouth gags (35) used for prolonged periods of time under anesthesia are a proposed risk factor for peri-anesthesia blindness and should be avoided. In a recent study, the blood flow to the retina through the maxillary artery was assessed in both the closed jaw position or upon maximal jaw opening with a spring-loaded metal mouth gag using computed tomography, electroretinography, and magnetic resonance angiography to measure perturbations in blood flow to the retina. Although blindness never occurred in these test subjects, alterations in blood flow to the retina through the maxillary artery was documented upon maximal jaw opening; therefore, any mouth gag, in particular spring-loaded metal mouth gags, should be used with great care, intermittently, and only for short durations, to minimize the risk of peri-anesthesia blindness.

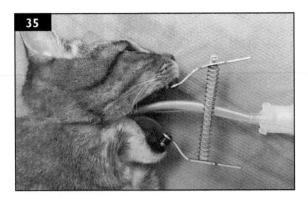

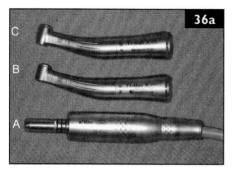

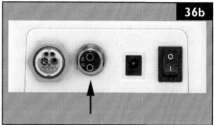

Question 36 This is a picture of an electric motor unit (**36a**, A) that has been retrofitted for use with a standard 4-hole dental line (**36b**, arrow) and a 1:5 E-type attachment (**36a**, C) that is comparable to a traditional air-driven high-speed handpiece. Electric motors and attachments are commonly used throughout Europe and Asia, but have been slow to take hold in the American marketplace. How does an electric attachment/motor differ from a traditional air-driven handpiece? What are the advantages and disadvantages of using an electric attachment?

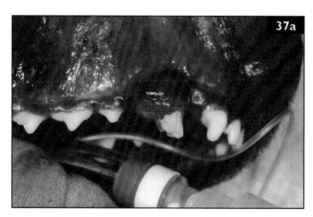

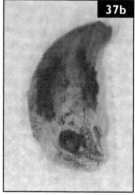

Question 37 This is a picture of a complicated crown-root fracture of the right maxillary canine tooth (**37a**) in a young dog. The tooth was treated by extraction, and there is a reddish growth of pulp tissue proliferating through the area of pulp exposure (**37b**). What is this growth?

36, 37: Answers

Answer 36 Compared to traditional air-driven high-speed handpieces that use a turbine and are low-torque instruments, electric motor attachments do not have a turbine, are gear driven, have a much higher torque, and do not experience as high a reduction in rpm when coming into contact with dental hard tissue. Electric motors can be operated in forward/reverse, have adjustable speeds and are significantly quieter in use (50 dB) than their air-driven counterparts. Electric attachments, however, are bulkier/heavier than air-driven high-speed handpieces, and are more expensive to purchase and maintain. Similar to lubed air-driven handpieces, electric attachments require lubrication after each use, and repeated autoclaving affects the longevity of the gear mechanism. Since electric attachments contain gears, the cost to replace these gears is considerably more expensive than replacing a turbine. Accidents such as the bur getting entangled with gauze or the patient's muzzle fur are both more expensive, but also more dangerous, since the electric motor will not stall when a bur becomes entangled, and will continue to spin at a constant rpm. In addition, the heat generated from the head of poorly maintained attachments may result in burns; third-degree burns have been reported in humans. Therefore, electric attachments must be maintained appropriately in accordance with manufacturer instructions to minimize this risk. Because they are gear driven, with rigid gear-to-gear contact and bearing support, burs are locked into position and there is no wobble or bur chatter. A typical electric motor runs at a maximum rpm of 40,000 rpm, and a 1:5 E-type attachment must be used to reach an rpm of 200,000 for comparable use to a traditional high-speed handpiece. When lower speeds are desired, the same motor can be used, but the 1:5 attachment is exchanged for a 1:1 E-type attachment (**36a, B**) that accepts RA latch-type burs, mandrels for abrasive discs, or drills such as a Gates-Glidden or Lentulo®. Essentially the purchase of only two different attachments is necessary for use with the one motor, and should allow one to perform all procedures, both high- and low-speed work.

Answer 37 This condition is referred to as a hyperplastic pulpitis where there is proliferative inflammation associated with an irreversible pulpitis, and is typically seen in carious lesions or in tooth fractures in immature animals where there is a generous blood supply or open apices. Epithelial cells in the saliva are implanted on the exposed pulp, resulting in a stratified squamous epithelial membrane or 'pulp polyp'. Although extraction was elected in this case, root canal treatment would also have been an excellent option.

Question 38 This is an intraoral view of the rostral maxillary region of an 11-year-old, spayed female cocker spaniel that was presented because of a 6-month history of chronic, purulent nasal discharge, severe halitosis and a large, progressive, painful swelling on the dorsal nasal region (38). Six months before this presentation, the left and right maxillary first and second incisor teeth were extracted and the remaining teeth were scaled and polished.

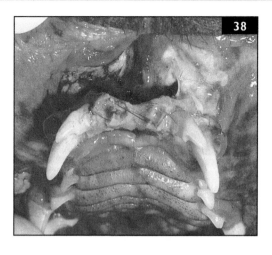

1 What is your tentative diagnosis, and what diagnostic tests are recommended to confirm your diagnosis?
2 Based on the results of further diagnostic testing, what is the diagnosis and appropriate treatment in this case?

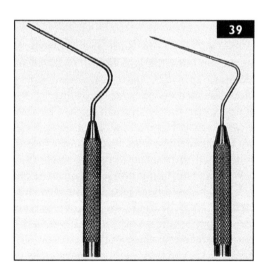

Question 39
1 What are the two instruments shown (39)?
2 What is the difference between them?
3 How are they each used?

41

Answer 38

1 Based on the history and the appearance of the lesion, osteonecrosis is suspected, although an underlying neoplastic process cannot be ruled out. Thoracic radiographs are necessary to reveal the presence of detectable metastatic disease. Hematologic and serum biochemical testing is recommended to rule out underlying disease; diagnostic imaging of the skull is recommended to further evaluate the lesion. An incisional biopsy followed by histopathologic examination is recommended to determine the exact nature of the condition.

The results of further diagnostic testing revealed normal thoracic radiographs and an elevated white blood cell count with a shift to the left. Skull radiographs revealed osteonecrosis in the region of the remaining maxillary incisor and canine teeth. Histopathologic examination revealed a severe chronic inflammatory reaction.

2 This is a case of osteonecrosis of the incisive bones. Appropriate treatment involves the removal of the necrotic bone and all remaining teeth associated with it. The surrounding bone is thoroughly débrided with rongeurs, curettes or surgical bur until normal, healthy bleeding bone is revealed. The excised tissue is submitted for histopathologic examination to confirm the diagnosis and tissue is submitted for bacterial culture and sensitivity testing. The surgical site is liberally flushed and the gingiva is sutured. Broad-spectrum antibiotic therapy is initiated pending the results of bacterial culture and sensitivity tests.

Answer 39

1 The instrument on the left is an endodontic *plugger* and the instrument on the right is an endodontic *spreader*. These instruments can come on long handles such as these, as double-ended instruments, or as finger instruments with a short working tip and a finger grip for use in small teeth. They come in various widths and lengths of the working tip. Heated versions of the spreaders are also available.
2 The plugger has a blunt end to the working tip and the spreader has the pointed tip.
3 The plugger is designed to push gutta-percha towards the apex during root canal obturation. With its blunt tip it presses against the gutta-percha and compacts it vertically. It can be used with heated gutta-percha placed into the canal and then compacted vertically, seating a single gutta-percha point apically or in true vertical condensation techniques where sized pluggers are used to compact sections of sized gutta-percha into the root canal.

The spreader is designed to compress gutta-percha laterally during obturation. The working tip can be warmed or used cold and is slid down alongside the gutta-percha to compact it laterally against the canal wall. Additional gutta-percha is placed either with warm gutta-percha techniques or using additional gutta-percha points that are again compacted laterally with the spreader. This process is repeated until the canal is completely filled. Using either or both instruments during root canal obturation creates a denser fill and can optimize filling irregularities in the canal.

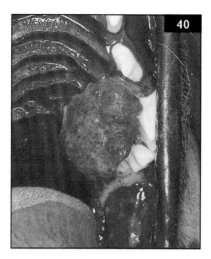

Question 40 This tumor on the caudal palate in a 7-year-old dog was diagnosed as a fibrosarcoma (**40**).
1 What are important factors in the therapeutic decision-making process?
2 Of what possible specific complications should the client be informed if a maxillectomy is considered?

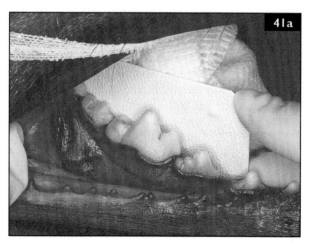

Question 41
1 What radiographic technique is being used here (**41a**) for obtaining a radiograph of the mandibular first molar tooth in a dog?
2 Where in the oral cavity can it be used?
3 Describe this technique.

40, 41: Answers

Answer 40

1 In addition to the general considerations of overall health, life expectancy, and wishes of the client, an accurate assessment of the extent of the tumor is extremely important. An oral fibrosarcoma infrequently has regional lymph node involvement and distant metastasis is occasionally present. Of particular importance in this case is to determine the extent of the primary tumor. Although good-quality oral and nasal radiographs may be useful, computed tomography is the diagnostic imaging modality of choice to establish the extent of the tumor as well as to assess regional lymph node involvement. Radiation therapy may be considered for remaining microscopic disease or if the extent of the tumor precludes surgical treatment.

2 The main intraoperative complication is hemorrhage, which can be life-threatening with inadequate anesthetic support and suboptimal surgical skill. Wide surgical margins are indicated as a fibrosarcoma is known to infiltrate deeply. Given the fact that this is a large tumor, tumor-free margins and tension-free closure may be difficult to achieve. The client should be informed that local recurrence is a distinct possibility. Partial dehiscence of the buccal flap used for closure of the maxillectomy site is generally due to closure under tension. The cheek on the operated side may be visibly pulled inwards. The mandibular teeth, the first molar tooth in particular, may occlude with and traumatize the flap covering the maxillectomy site.

Answer 41

1 The parallel technique, which is one of the two basic intraoral radiographic techniques (**41b**).

2 The parallel technique is a very accurate technique but it can only be used if the dental film can be placed parallel to the tooth, which may be difficult due to the shape of the oral cavity. Using intraorally placed dental films, the only teeth that allow film placement parallel to their roots are the caudal mandibular premolar and molar teeth in the dog and the premolar and molar teeth in the cat. A near-parallel technique is also used for the extraoral view of the maxillary premolar and molar teeth in the cat.

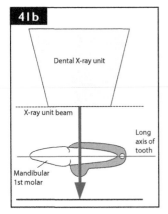

3 The intraoral film packet is placed parallel to the tooth being radiographed. The plane of the film should be parallel to the plane of the tooth. The central X-ray beam is directed perpendicular to the structure being radiographed and the film. If one notices that a slight angle is formed by the tooth and the film, a satisfactory film will be produced by directing the central X-ray beam perpendicular to the tooth. If the angle is greater than 15°, then a bisecting angle technique should be used (see **190**). The radiographic image will be elongated if the bisecting angle technique is not used.

Question 42 Conscious oral examination of a 4-year-old, castrated male Maine Coon cat (42) revealed periodontal disease and tooth resorption lesions. The remainder of the physical examination was unremarkable with the exception of a Grade II–III/VI systolic murmur, best heard parasternally, and a gallop rhythm. The cat was strictly 'indoors' and fairly inactive, and the clients did not notice any respiratory or behavioral changes.

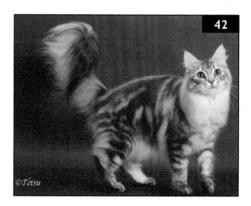

1 What is your assessment of the findings found on cardiac auscultation?
2 What diagnostic testing would you recommend before general anesthesia?

Question 43 In this 7-month-old dog, the deciduous canine tooth is still in place and not mobile (43). It is fractured and a draining tract is visible overlying the root tip (arrow). What is the treatment of choice, and why?

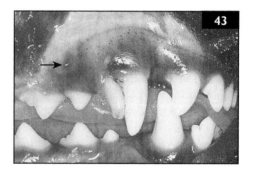

Question 44 What areas of the oral cavity are affected by stomatitis in this cat (44)?

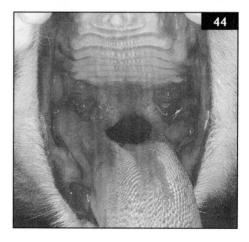

Answer 42

1 Based on the signalment, history, and physical examination, hypertrophic cardiomyopathy (HCM) is the most likely diagnosis. Systolic anterior motion of the mitral valve causing mitral valve regurgitation and partial left ventricular outflow tract obstruction from septal hypertrophy are common causes of the heart murmur in HCM cats. The gallop rhythm indicates ventricular diastolic dysfunction which is commonly seen in cats with cardiomyopathy. Cardiomyopathy is the most common heart condition in cats. More than 50% of cats with HCM exhibit few to no symptoms at the time of presentation. Thirty percent of Maine Coon cats have a mutation in the cardiac myosin-binding protein C gene which has been associated with a higher risk of developing HCM. Genetic tests for this gene mutation are available.

2 A complete blood count, biochemical profile, including thyroid hormone tests, and urinalysis should be performed. A cardiac evaluation is required to diagnose the cardiac disorder and to determine appropriate treatment. The cardiac evaluation could include an electrocardiogram, thoracic radiographs, Doppler blood pressure measurements and an echocardiogram. An echocardiogram is required to diagnose the presence and form of cardiomyopathy. Although HCM is strongly suspected in this case, cats can also have dilated cardiomyopathy, and the two conditions must be differentiated from one another. The anesthesia and dental care should be delayed until the cardiac disorder has been diagnosed and appropriately managed. The potential for complications associated with anesthesia should be evaluated and discussed with the clients. Appropriate adjustments in anesthetic protocols should be made based on the underlying cardiac disease. The clinician should be prepared to manage complications that may occur during anesthesia as well as during recovery and the days following anesthesia.

Answer 43 Extraction should be performed immediately. Resorption of deciduous teeth is dependent on the presence of living cells (odontoclasts). In this case, these cells were destroyed due to pulp necrosis resulting from the complicated fracture and subsequent periapical pathology (draining tract). The raised opening of the draining tract is known as a 'parulis'. Any resorptive activity ceased, causing the deciduous canine tooth to stay in place. If the fractured deciduous tooth remains in place for a long period of time, the infection can easily spread further and cause a local osteomyelitis as well as affecting the permanent canine tooth.

Answer 44 Stomatitis refers to inflammation of the oral mucosa, and different areas may be affected. In this case the palatoglossal folds and the areas lateral to them, the caudal part of the oral cavity proper, are affected. Inflammation of this area has previously incorrectly been referred to as 'faucitis'. However, the fauces are located medial to the palatoglossal folds, not lateral. In this case there is also gingivitis present in the areas where full-mouth extractions were performed.

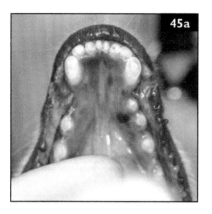
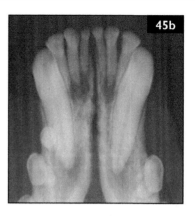

Question 45 A 5-year-old male Chihuahua was presented with a history of intermittent jaw chattering and dropping kibble from his mouth. This picture (45a) was obtained under anesthesia; conscious oral examination was not possible due to the patient's aggressive disposition. The client-provided patient history included failed attempts at behavioral modification for human-directed aggression.
1 Describe the radiographic findings in this intraoral mandibular occlusal view radiograph (45b) obtained in this patient.
2 What is the most likely cause for the dental condition identified in this patient?

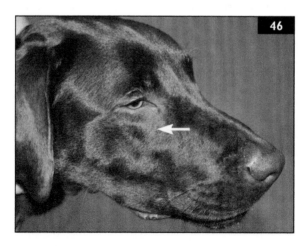

Question 46 This patient was presented for evaluation of bilateral swellings rostroventral to the eyes (46, arrow). The swellings are periodic and do not appear to be associated with regional or distant disease. What are these swellings?

Answer 45

1 The left mandibular first premolar tooth is missing and the right mandibular second premolar tooth is single-rooted. There are well-defined periapical radiolucencies associated with the mandibular incisor and canine teeth consistent with chronic periapical periodontitis. The cusp tips of the mandibular canine teeth are missing.

2 In addition to the findings on clinical and radiographic examination, review of the patient's medical records revealed that a 'canine disarming' procedure was performed several years ago, where the incisor and canine teeth were deliberately shortened in height to address the patient's aggression. 'Canine disarming', where either strategic crown-height reduction or extractions are performed as a treatment for aggression, is a controversial procedure, whose proponents report improvement in the patient's demeanor and less trauma to those that are bitten when this procedure is performed. Behavioral modification, with or without pharmaceutical treatment, remains the standard of care for dog aggression, and consultation with a board-certified veterinary behavior specialist is recommended. The clients were unaware of the radiographic follow-up necessary with this procedure when the procedure is performed correctly, or of the damage incurred to non-diseased teeth, especially if the procedure is performed incorrectly. When teeth are 'disarmed', shortened in height as in this case, the pulp cavity is exposed; in doing so either vital pulp therapy or standard root canal therapy must be performed. In the radiograph (45b), evidence of an endodontic procedure is not present; therefore either endodontic therapy was never performed, or through abrasion, the patient wore through the restorative material and exposed the pulp, resulting in pulpitis and subsequent pulp necrosis. Surgical extraction of the infected teeth was recommended.

Answer 46 These nodular swellings are the buccal lymph nodes (*lymphonodi buccales*), which are infrequently (9% of dogs) present unilaterally or bilaterally, located dorsal to the zygomatic muscle and rostral to the masseter muscle in the region where the superior labial vein drains into the facial vein (i.e. angle of confluence). Their location is variable with respect to the facial vein. The buccal lymph nodes are flattened nodules, variable in size (approximately 10 mm × 5 mm), and may be seen more frequently in larger purebred dogs. Besides the dog, these nodes have also been described in humans, primates, rabbits, guinea pigs, camels, and rats. Because of their location, these nodes must be distinguished from other regionally located anatomy such as the ventral buccal salivary gland, accessory parotid gland, and infection-related suborbital swellings (e.g. periapical disease of the maxillary fourth premolar tooth). Although enlargement of the buccal lymph nodes may be associated with regional disease (upper lip) or distant disease (metastasis), the drainage of these nodes remains poorly described, and in some cases their enlargement is idiopathic.

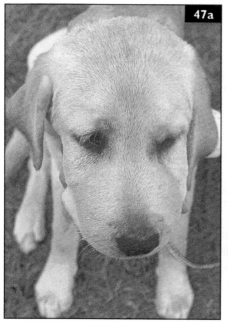
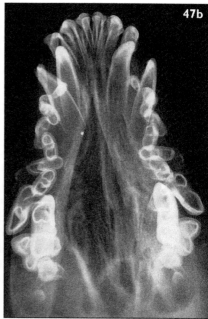

Question 47
1 What is the primary differential diagnosis in this 8-month-old dog on a balanced diet (**47a, b**)?
2 What is the mechanism for the development of this problem?

Question 48 The most important aspect of atraumatic extraction technique is the severing of the periodontal ligament, which is most frequently performed using dental luxators and elevators.
1 What are the main differences between dental elevators and luxators?
2 Why are elevators and luxators produced in different sizes and tip curvatures?

47, 48: Answers

Answer 47

1 Renal secondary hyperparathyroidism. Radiologic changes in renal secondary hyperparathyroidism include generalized bone loss with a greater extent of loss occurring in the bones of the skull. The bones of the head are affected before involvement of the axial skeleton or long bones. The mandible is affected first followed by the bones in the maxilla. The earliest radiologic evidence of bone loss is loss of the lamina dura (the radiologically apparent radiopaque line surrounding the tooth roots; see 77); bone loss continues in the interdental and interradicular regions with severe cortical bone loss eventually occurring.

2 The skeletal changes occur secondary to chronic renal insufficiency, which results in secondary hyperparathyroidism. The 'classic explanation' is that phosphorus retention occurs as the kidneys progressively lose their ability to excrete phosphorus; phosphorus retention decreases extracellular calcium due to the mass law equation; the parathyroids are chronically stimulated to maintain extracellular calcium concentration within the normal range. An alternative theory has been proposed, namely the 'vitamin D trade-off hypothesis.' According to this theory there is a decrease in vitamin D synthesis in the proximal renal tubules; decreased serum vitamin D levels result in loss of negative feedback on the parathyroid gland; decreased serum vitamin D levels also result in a decreased serum calcium level; an increase in serum parathyroid hormone (PTH) level occurs as a result of decreased serum vitamin D and calcium.

Answer 48

1 Dental elevators are fashioned with a cutting edge in chisel form while luxators are more knife-like. Elevators are made from hardened metal and are robust instruments which can withstand heavy handling. They are sharpened in the form of a chisel and often also go under that name. Luxators are produced from softer metal which can be readily sharpened. The thin, highly-tapered tip of a luxator (48 bottom) penetrates the narrow periodontal space far more readily than the 'chunky' tip of an elevator (48 top). When used appropriately, mechanical advantage reduces the effort required to do the work of extraction. Luxators have a thin, tapered blade which can be used as an efficient gradient wedge.

2 The width and curvature of the instrument tips need to conform to the roots of the teeth on which they are used, so a wide variety of sizes is required. For veterinary

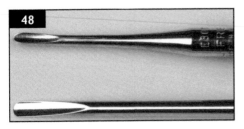

use the most common sizes are 2, 3, 4, and 5 mm, the larger three sizes being standard sizes used by human dentists. Various manufacturers interpret the designs differently, so by shopping around it is possible to obtain a set of instruments to suit all small animal dental needs.

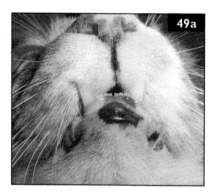
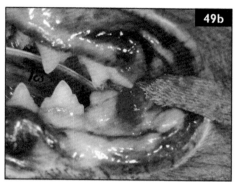

Question 49 These cats recently had extractions of both maxillary canine teeth (49a) and the left mandibular first molar tooth (49b).
1 What postoperative complication has developed in both cats?
2 How is this condition treated?

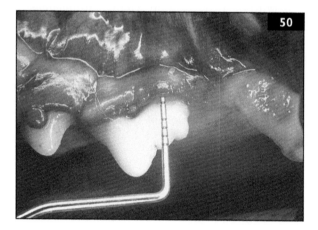

Question 50 This maxillary second premolar tooth (50) has a measured probing depth (pocket depth) of 5 mm with 2–3 mm of gingival recession around the distal root.
1 What is the attachment loss around the distal root?
2 What is the significance of this attachment loss for this tooth?

51

49, 50: Answers

Answer 49

1 Traumatic occlusion following tooth extraction is a complication typically limited to the cat, where there is an injurious occlusion of an opposing tooth into the oral soft tissues after a tooth has been extracted, usually following extraction of the mandibular first molar tooth, or in the case of the extracted maxillary canine tooth, where the opposing mandibular canine tooth becomes entrapped extraoral to the maxillary lip, resulting in ulceration or even puncture injury of the lip. Loss of the clinical height of the maxillary canine tooth results in an infolding of the upper lip causing the entrapment with the mandibular canine tooth, particularly in brachycephalic cat breeds or cat breeds such as the Siamese cat, which have a triangular or wedge-shaped face. Injury to the intraoral soft tissues, particularly to the vestibular mucogingival tissues of the mandibular first molar tooth, ranges from ulceration (indentation of the cusp tip in the mucosa) to development of mucosal polyp formation or pyogenic granuloma, which may easily be mistaken in clinical appearance for neoplasia.

2 If the patient shows the ability to self-correct the lip entrapment, and there is no soft-tissue trauma, treatment is not indicated. If, however, the maxillary lip is swollen secondary to the extraction procedure, anti-inflammatory medications may be successful in reducing the swelling, and the entrapment may resolve uneventfully once the swelling subsides. Conservative odontoplasty, blunting of the cusp tip of the offending tooth using a dental finishing bur without entry into the pulp chamber, may rectify the traumatic malocclusion in mild cases. In more severe cases, crown-height reduction of the mandibular canine tooth followed by vital pulp therapy or standard root canal treatment may be indicated, and at last resort, extraction of the offending tooth or teeth may be performed.

Answer 50

1 The attachment loss around the distal root of this premolar tooth is 7–8 mm.

2 Probing depth (pocket depth) measures the distance from the apical limit of the pocket to the free gingival margin. A sulcus depth of 3 mm or less is normal in a dog, while the cat has a normal sulcus of 1 mm or less. A probing depth of 5 mm indicates there is the beginning of periodontal disease with the loss of periodontal ligament attachment to the root cementum. Gingival recession is where the free gingival margin moves apically from the cementoenamel junction (CEJ). When there is gingival recession along with an increased probing depth this shows there is even greater periodontal ligament loss and bone loss around this tooth and/or root. The combination of the gingival recession measurement and the probing depth is called the attachment loss. It provides a more accurate measurement of the periodontal health status of a tooth.

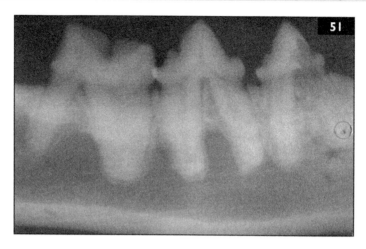

Question 51 What radiographic abnormalities can you see in the mandible of this cat (**51**)?

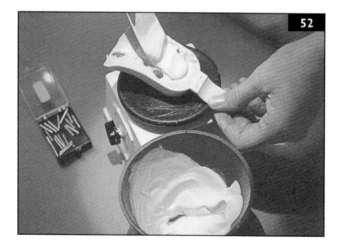

Question 52
1 What are the important considerations regarding time and pouring for alginate and vinyl polysiloxane impressions (**52**)?
2 How can air bubbles be avoided when pouring a stone model?

51, 52: Answers

Answer 51 The third premolar tooth has a clinically evident feline tooth resorption (TR) lesion at its buccal gingival margin. The radiograph demonstrates severe radiographic changes – there is root and crown resorption (seen as sharp-edged, but irregular areas of radiolucency) and ankylosis, affecting primarily the mesial root, consistent with a type-3 lesion. Note that the fourth premolar tooth is normal. Radiographs often delineate the extent of the resorption more accurately than clinical examination alone (often the clinical lesion is only the tip of the iceberg), and no TR should be treated without prior radiographic examination. Teeth with resorptive lesions rarely lose their endodontic blood supply, so pulp necrosis followed by a clinically or radiographically evident periapical lesion is unusual. Lesions that are evident at the gingival margin often have some periodontal bone loss and loss of attachment, or there may be concurrent periodontal disease. This third premolar tooth is typical of the radiographic features of feline TR lesions.

Answer 52
1 *Alginate impressions*: the stone models should be poured within 30 minutes, unless one of the newer alginates that remain stable for a longer period of time is used. Excess water should be removed from alginate impressions. If the stone model is not poured immediately, the impression should be wrapped in a dampened paper towel and kept in the refrigerator. After 24 hours, discard the impression.

Vinyl polysiloxane impressions: delay the stone model pouring for 1 hour in order to obtain the best surface on the model (small gas bubbles may come to the surface during the first hour). Pouring may be delayed up to 14 days without loss of accuracy.

2 Wet the stone in the center of the mixing bowl by stirring with a spatula. Once the stone is wet, begin spatulating it on the side of the mixing bowl. Spatulate in one direction to minimize air bubbles. The bowl can be placed on the vibrator to remove any air bubbles. The mixing time should be less than 2 minutes. One end of the impression is placed on the vibrator and small amounts of dental stone are placed at the opposite end of the impression. The vibration will cause the stone to flow into the impression. The flow should be controlled to avoid air being trapped in the deep recesses of the impressions. Once the teeth and floor of the impression have been carefully filled with stone, the vibrator is turned off and small brass pins (Pindex®, Coltène/Whaledent Inc., Cuyahoga Falls, OH) are gently inserted into the canine teeth so that only the tips of the pins appear from the stone. The remainder of the stone is thickened and added to the top of the model. It is important to build up the model to strengthen it. The model is then placed on a level surface to allow the initial set to occur which takes approximately 10–15 minutes. The mixing and pouring of the dental stone should be done in less than 5 minutes. After 45–60 minutes the impression can be separated from the stone model.

Question 53 The appropriate management of traumatic lesions of lips in dogs and cats varies depending on the clinical presentation (53).

1 What should be included in the initial wound management of lip lacerations?
2 What factors influence whether or not a lip laceration should be closed primarily or closed utilizing delayed primary closure?

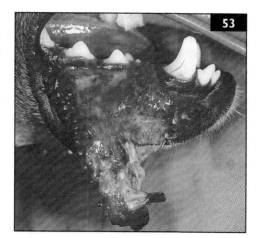

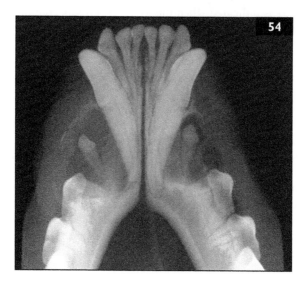

Question 54 The intraoral examination of an 18-month-old Shih Tzu revealed two 15 mm, smooth, soft, non-painful, fluctuating swellings in the edentulous areas distal to the mandibular canine teeth and mesial to the mandibular second premolar teeth. Aspiration of the swelling produced a serous, slightly blood-tinged fluid. Intraoral radiographs were taken of the rostral mandible (54).

1 What is your tentative diagnosis?
2 What is the appropriate treatment for this condition?
3 What complications may be encountered in the management of this patient?

Answer 53

1 Initial wound management should include débridement of devitalized tissue and copious lavage. The condition of the wound following débridement will influence the decision on timing and method of wound closure.

2 Several factors influencing primary wound closure include: degree of contamination, time interval since injury, presence of devitalized and damaged tissue, adequacy of blood supply, availability of tension-free closure, overall status of the patient, and client compliance with wound management. Acute wounds can usually be débrided and closed primarily, which is the preferred method. A full-thickness lip laceration should be closed in two layers. The mucosa is apposed with simple-interrupted absorbable sutures with the knots located within the oral cavity, while the skin is apposed with simple-interrupted non-absorbable sutures. In general, the number of sutures should be kept to a minimum. The suture size should be as small as possible; usually 5-0 suture material is adequate and the sutures should be carefully placed, taking care not to devitalize tissues. Delayed primary closure is indicated when the wound is grossly contaminated, purulent, extensively devitalized, edematous, or inflamed. Delayed primary closure is performed 3–5 days after injury. The advantage of delayed primary closure is that it permits evaluation of the progression of wound healing and serial débridement of devitalized tissue, but it may result in a more prominent scar.

Answer 54

1 Bilateral dentigerous cysts, containing unerupted mandibular first premolar teeth. Although dentigerous cysts occur infrequently in dogs, it should be a primary consideration in young dogs presented with oral swellings in an edentulous area.

2 Treatment involves making an incision over the cyst, burring away any buccal cortical bone overlying the cyst, drainage of fluid, and extraction of the unerupted tooth following minimal elevation. The cyst wall is thoroughly curetted to ensure complete removal. The entire cyst lining should be submitted for histopathologic examination. The use of a cancellous bone graft is recommended. The oral mucosa is closed with multiple, simple-interrupted sutures.

3 Incomplete removal of the cystic epithelium may result in recurrence of the dentigerous cyst. Malignant transformation of the epithelial lining cells of the dentigerous cyst to primary osseous carcinoma, adenomatoid odontogenic tumor, and ameloblastoma has been reported in humans; this potential, although rare, exists in dogs, making thorough histopathologic examination and careful postoperative evaluation of the surgical site mandatory. The structure of the mandible will be considerably weakened as a result of the cysts and surgery, and care should be taken to avoid fracture of the mandible.

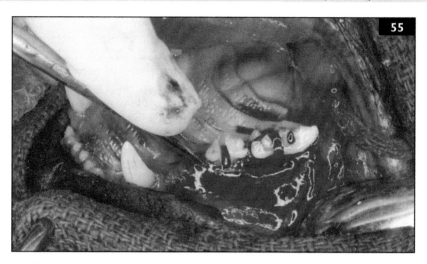

Question 55 Full-mouth extraction is an accepted surgical option for patients with chronic gingivostomatitis (**55**).
1 What does the procedure encompass?
2 Describe your immediate postoperative regimen for these patients.

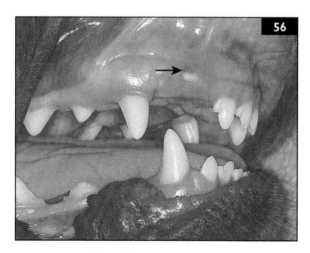

Question 56 This 6-month-old dog exfoliated the deciduous dentition in time and the permanent dentition is in place. Only the tip of the crown of the maxillary third incisor tooth is visible through the gingiva (**56**, arrow). What is your diagnosis, and what is the recommended treatment?

Answer 55

1 Extracting all teeth (full mouth), possibly with the exception of the canine and incisor teeth (partial mouth). In a recent study, no significant difference in overall response to treatment was found between cats treated by partial-mouth versus full-mouth extractions. Although extraction therapy alone may result in satisfactory clinical improvement in many cats, concurrent long-term medical therapy is often necessary to achieve substantial improvement or cure.

It is essential that the whole tooth, i.e. crown and root(s), is completely removed. The least traumatic means of doing this is surgical extraction using a flap technique. Preoperative radiographs are always indicated. Following extraction, radiographs should be performed to ensure that there are no root remnants. Any remaining root fragments should be removed before flap closure.

Extractions should be completed one quadrant at a time. A mucogingival flap is raised to expose the furcations and buccal bone plate of the premolar teeth and molar teeth. Multirooted teeth are sectioned into single-rooted segments using a bur in either a high-speed or low-speed handpiece. Buccal bone is also removed with the bur to facilitate extraction. Water cooling of the bur is mandatory. Enough bone should be removed to allow easy extraction yet trying to maintain as much as possible of the alveolar bone height. The teeth are then gently elevated or luxated out of their alveoli. Gentle curettage of the vacated alveoli and alveoloplasty should be performed to ensure a smooth alveolar margin. The mucogingival flap is repositioned and sutured tension-free.

2 The immediate postoperative consideration is analgesia. Cats which have had full four-quadrant extraction are usually uncomfortable. Pre-emptive analgesia, including opioids or other analgesics, and regional anesthetic blocks will provide pain relief for a few hours after recovery, and may be indicated for a longer period postoperatively. An esophagostomy feeding tube may be indicated in severe cases for nutritional support. In some instances, it is useful to stage the surgery, i.e. extract the maxillary and mandibular teeth on one side on the first occasion, and then do the other side a few weeks later, or extract the premolar and molar teeth first, to be followed by the incisor and canine teeth later.

Answer 56 The third incisor tooth is retained and embedded. Radiographs are indicated to visualize the position and morphology of this tooth. Extraction is the treatment of choice. Most of the crown is located subgingivally. The gingiva does not attach to the enamel surface, except at the epithelial attachment at the most apical part of the crown. The result is a deep gingival pseudopocket, which will trap bacteria, food, and debris, leading to pericoronitis. Extraction should be performed as soon as possible. Orthodontic treatment of this condition is impractical and not in the interest of the patient. This displaced tooth has to be extruded and possibly moved and tipped. Although this is possible and is standard treatment in human orthodontics, the treatment would require a very difficult series of different appliances and a long treatment period.

Question 57 What radiographic error is evident on the radiograph in question 51?

Question 58 An 8-year-old, spayed female Labrador retriever was presented for traumatic malocclusion associated with mandibular drift following a left segmental mandibulectomy that was performed to treat a canine acanthomatous ameloblastoma. Crown-height reduction with vital pulp therapy had been performed on both mandibular canines at the time of the mandibulectomy (58a) in an attempt to avoid this complication; however, oral examination 1-week postoperative revealed traumatic occlusion of the left maxillary canine tooth into the lingual mucosa (58b).

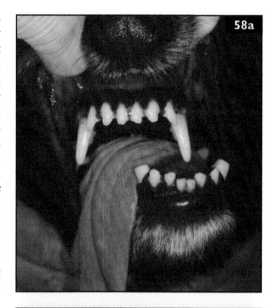

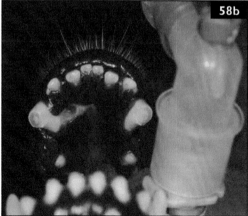

1 Define mandibular drift. When should mandibular drift be anticipated?
2 What are conservative treatment alternatives to extraction or crown-height reduction following mandibulectomy?

57, 58: Answers

Answer 57 The embossed dot on conventional radiograph film is superimposed on the apical part of the mesial root of the third premolar tooth. This is a common error in radiographic positioning. The dot can obliterate subtle lesions or be falsely diagnosed as a pathologic lesion. When positioning the film in the oral cavity, the dot, or any other marker on a digital system, should be located away from structures of potential interest, such as the roots, and rather be placed where there is no overlap with dental structures. This does not affect the use of the embossed dot in orienting radiographs (see **199**).

Answer 58
1 Mandibular drift is defined as the lingual (medial) displacement of the intact mandible caused by destabilization of the lower jaw structure and the action of the medial pterygoid muscle following mandibulectomy, and should be an anticipated complication when performing segmental mandibulectomy and total unilateral mandibulectomy.
2 Although reconstruction following mandibular resection surgery is the ideal solution to preventing mandibular drift, access to facilities performing such advanced surgeries is currently limited. As an alternative to more invasive and facially disfiguring procedures such as surgical extraction or crown-height reduction that only treat the painful malocclusion caused by the drift, elastic training of the muscles of mastication is a preferable non-invasive technique. This technique uses an elastomeric chain attached between orthodontic buttons that have been cemented to the lingual surface of the mandibular canine tooth and buccal surface of the maxillary fourth premolar tooth (**58c, d**) of the intact mandible to train the medial pterygoid muscle to resist the lingual pull in the direction of the resected mandible. The chain is replaced at a minimum of weekly, and is used in this fashion until the normal canine occlusion resumes, in roughly 4–6 months. Variations of this muscular training technique in terms of anchorage location and materials are limited only by the creativity of the surgeon; traditional maxillomandibular fixation screws (**58e**) or orthodontic temporary anchorage devices, are suitable alternatives to orthodontic buttons.

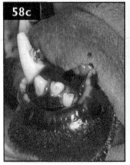 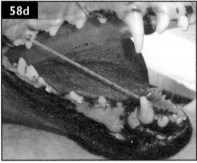 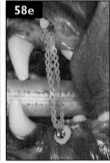

Question 59 The eosinophilic granuloma complex in cats refers to a group of lesions affecting the skin and oral cavity (59). Oral eosinophilic granulomas also occur in dogs.

1 Which lesions affect cats, and where are they typically located?

2 In which breeds of dog are these lesions most common, and where do they usually occur in the oral cavity?

3 What are the recommended treatment options?

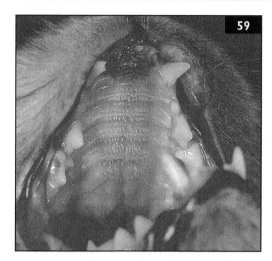

Question 60 A 6-year-old Rottweiler with a history of moderate subaortic stenosis (60) was presented for professional dental cleaning and extraction of multiple fractured teeth with pulp exposure. At present, there is no reported exercise intolerance, but there is a history of syncope, and the patient does receive a beta blocker.

1 What is a potential severe complication associated with performing dental therapy in this patient?

2 What treatment is recommended to reduce the risk of this complication?

3 What other disease conditions require the same treatment?

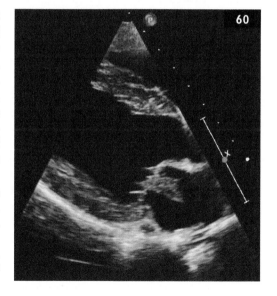

59, 60: Answers

Answer 59

1 Oral lesions in cats are usually eosinophilic ulcers or linear granulomas. Eosinophilic ulcers (e.g. indolent, rodent, and lip ulcers) are non-painful, non-pruritic lesions most commonly found on the upper lip. They are usually well-circumscribed, firm, red-brown to yellow, ulcerated lesions located on each side of the midline (59). Eosinophilic granulomas (linear granulomas) may occur as single or multiple lesions in a nodular pattern in the oral cavity. Histologic evaluation of these oral lesions is necessary for definitive diagnosis and to differentiate them from neoplasms, mycotic infections, and foreign body reactions.

2 An eosinophilic granuloma may occur in any breed but occurs most commonly in young Siberian huskies. These lesions are typically identified as proliferative tissue, with or without superficial ulcerations, located primarily on the lateral and ventral surfaces of the tongue. Eosinophilic stomatitis mainly occurs in the cavalier King Charles spaniel and is characterized by plaques in the oropharynx and on the soft palate, which may be asymptomatic or cause dysphagia.

3 Whenever possible an underlying etiology such as allergies should be identified and treated. Lesions may regress spontaneously. In symptomatic cases lesions generally respond to a short to medium course of anti-inflammatory glucocorticoid treatment. Surgical treatment is rarely indicated.

Answer 60

1 Infective (bacterial) endocarditis.

2 Prophylactic antibiotics are recommended prior to dental surgery in dogs with subaortic stenosis to reduce the risk of bacterial endocarditis. Penicillin is often recommended as the antibiotic of choice for this purpose; however, the sufficiency of its spectrum is questionable, and broader coverage with the addition of a fluoroquinolone or metronidazole may be warranted.

3 In contrast, dogs with myxomatous mitral valve degeneration are not considered at high risk for bacterial endocarditis, and the use of prophylactic antibiotics prior to professional dental cleaning in these dogs is not currently recommended. Moreover, the signalment of dogs with mitral valve disease is typically the small-breed dog, compared to the signalment of the dog with infective endocarditis, which is often the medium- to large-breed purebred dog, further debunking the myth that prophylactic antibiotics are recommended for all dogs with heart murmurs. At present, the current recommendations for prophylactic antibiotic (1 hour before the procedure) usage in dogs with dental procedures, to reduce the risk of the associated bacteremia resulting in secondary bacterial endocarditis, as adapted from the current human guidelines, include patients with previous infective endocarditis, prosthetic valves, or congenital outflow tract cardiac disease (e.g. subaortic stenosis). Although complete adherence to these recommendations is challenging, and certainly clinical judgment must be used on a case-by-case basis, adopting a judicious approach to antibiotic usage, in general, is an important step towards reducing antibiotic resistance.

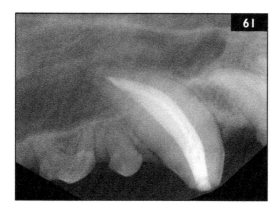

Question 61 This is a procedural radiograph of root canal therapy of a canine tooth (**61**).
1 Evaluate the quality of the root canal fill.
2 Why is a good obturation of the apical third of a root canal important?

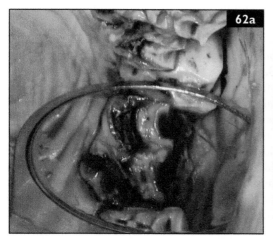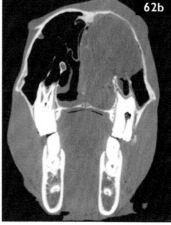

Question 62 This horse was presented for a left-sided nasal discharge. Photograph (**62a**) and computed tomography (CT) image (**62b**) is provided at the level of the left maxillary first molar tooth.
1 Can the nasal discharge be explained by a dental condition?
2 What treatment is indicated?
3 What are the complications of tooth repulsion?

61, 62: Answers

Answer 61

1 Although the coronal two-thirds of the canal have a dense fill, the apical third has a poorly compacted fill.

2 Although a dense fill in the coronal two-thirds (along with the access restorations) would prevent contamination of the apex from materials in the oral cavity, apical voids may cause eventual failure, even in a well-cleaned canal. If a space exists between the root canal obturating material and the dentin, percolation of fluids can occur. Residual bacteria, bacterial breakdown products, toxins, or organic debris in the canal can act as periapical tissue irritants. Even in a well-cleaned canal, fluid ingress from periapical tissues can stagnate in microvoids in the canal. Fluid breakdown products can then diffuse back out, acting as an irritant. A third source of potential problems is the seeding of bacteria from transient bacteremia causing reinfection of a previously non-infected canal. In carnivores, most of the teeth on which root canal therapy is performed have an apical delta rather than a large apical foramen. An apical delta consists of many small canals at the apex (see 66). In endodontic therapy, good technique achieves a three-dimensional fill to treat and obturate all the portals of exit (POE), including any lateral canals. An apical delta can be visualized as a high concentration of tiny 'lateral' canals in the apical 1–4 mm of the root. A small 'blush' of sealant from the apical POEs indicates a treated and well-filled apex.

Answer 62

1 The left maxillary first molar tooth has a complicated crown–root fracture with exposure of pulp horns 3, 4, and 5. The CT image shows a soft-tissue-like density of the sinus cavities. This was found to be inspissated purulent material. The endodontic failure of the left maxillary first molar tooth has allowed bacteria to invade the sinus compartments and a secondary sinusitis to develop.

2 Treatment would include extraction of the tooth performed via an oral approach. Oral approach could include minimal invasive buccotomy due to the diseased clinical crown forbidding delivery with forceps. Sinus trephination, evacuation of the purulent material and lavage of the sinus compartments would be performed to treat the secondary sinusitis. To protect against chronic fistula formation, repulsion of the tooth should be avoided.

3 The complications which can occur at the time of repulsion or shortly thereafter include: (1) Traumatic fracture. (2) Iatrogenic damage to neighboring teeth. (3) Inadvertent disruption of adjacent structures: nasolacrimal duct; parotid salivary duct; branches of the linguofacial artery and vein; palatine artery; ventral and dorsal buccal branches of the facial nerve; infraorbital nerve. (4) Failure to remove the entire tooth – dental sequestration. (5) Sequestration of bone fragments from the lining of the alveolus. (6) Loss of the alveolar plug with contamination of the alveolus by ingesta. (7) Oronasal fistula formation.

Diseased teeth that can be associated with secondary sinusitis include the maxillary fourth premolar tooth, first molar, second molar, and third molar teeth.

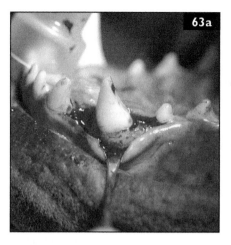 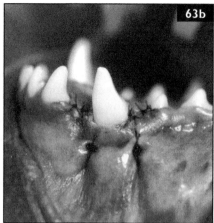

Question 63

1 Which procedure is being performed on this dog's maxillary canine tooth (63a, b)?
2 What technique would be indicated?

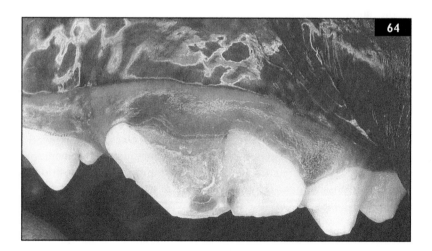

Question 64

1 Classify this type of tooth fracture (64) according to the American Veterinary Dental College (AVDC) nomenclature classification of dental fractures.
2 What are the treatment objectives indicated?

Answer 63

1 Due to the depth of the fracture and the size of the remaining crown, a crown-lengthening procedure must be performed.

2 A type I crown-lengthening involves a gingivectomy and would be insufficient. A type II crown-lengthening is performed here. An incision along the sulcus is made from the borders of adjacent teeth. Releasing incisions are made at adjacent teeth. The gingiva is reflected away from the bone and tooth with a periosteal elevator, exposing the bone. Marginal alveolar bone is removed to increase the coronal length. A conventional crown preparation is performed. Impressions are obtained. At this point, the gingiva is sutured to its new apically relocated position. A type III crown-lengthening would be orthodontic extrusion, which is more indicated for unerupted teeth.

Answer 64

1 This is a complicated crown–root fracture. The 'complicated' refers to the fact that pulp exposure has occurred, and 'crown–root' to the fact that enamel, dentin, and cementum are involved in the fracture line. This type of fracture by definition extends under the level of the gingiva and may extend under the level of the alveolar margin. The term 'slab fracture' is commonly used for this type of fracture but does not specifically imply pulp exposure or subgingival involvement. In this particular case, the pulp is considered vital because there is still some bleeding evident.

2 The primary treatment objectives (if conservative treatment is elected) are to prevent endodontic disease caused by the pulp exposure, and periodontal disease caused by the distortion of the normal gingival contour. An additional treatment objective may be to restore the normal morphology of the tooth.

Crown–root fractures involve the periodontal ligament and may lead to periodontitis because of the altered gingival contour. A small fracture fragment and the overlying unsupported gingiva can be removed to restore a physiologic contour. A fracture extending under the level of the alveolar margin may be treated by creating a periodontal flap (see 173), removing the fracture fragment, performing an osteoplasty, and repositioning the flap in a more apical position. Crown restoration is possible provided the furcation is not involved, and may help in restoring the gingival contour. The restoration should ideally include the re-creation of the tooth bulge coronal to the cementoenamel junction. This can help to prevent further periodontal problems caused by food entrapment into the void that was created by the loss of tooth substance. A prosthetic crown may also be used to restore the gingival contour and to protect the tooth from further trauma (see 143). Deep crown–root fractures lead to an irreversible periodontitis and are an indication for extraction.

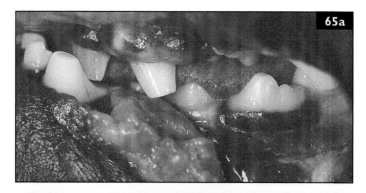

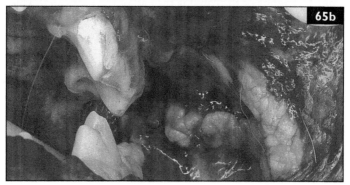

Question 65

1 Seen here are two examples of what condition in the dog (65a, b)?
2 Where else in the oral cavity may lesions of similar origin be found?
3 What is the recommended treatment?

Question 66 The root apex of the tooth is the tip of the root (66a).

1 What are the anatomic landmarks of this area in humans?
2 How does the apical morphology differ in dogs and cats compared with humans?
3 What is the clinical relevance of this morphologic feature?

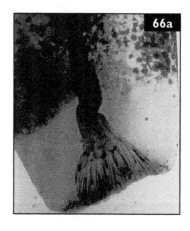

65, 66: Answers

Answer 65

1 These are examples of labial and buccal mucosal hyperplasia of self-inflicted, traumatic origin, commonly known as 'gum-chewing lesions'. Originally described in small, excessively barking dog breeds, it may be found in other breeds, as well as in cats.

2 Excessive loose mucosal folds and indurated hyperplastic mucosa may also be found sublingually.

3 Surgical excision is indicated in selected cases. Resected tissue should be submitted for histopathologic examination to confirm the diagnosis and exclude neoplasia.

Answer 66

1 The apical terminus of the canal is the end of the root canal which is synonymous with the apical constriction, the narrowest diameter of the canal. The foramen is the opening created by the canal ending on the external root surface. There is a funnel-shaped space between the apical constriction internal to the foramen and the foramen on the external root surface (**66b**). The cementum invaginates inside this cone and ends at the cementodentinal junction (CDJ) at or close to the apical constriction. The CDJ delimitates where pulp becomes periapical tissue.

2 In humans, the apical area is composed of a principal foramen with sometimes a few smaller accessory foramina. In dogs and cats, a complex apical delta is a normal feature of the apex of mature teeth. Between 10 and 20 foramina are seen in dogs' and cats' canine teeth and the apical ramifications connecting the apical terminus to the foramina are 1.75–2 mm long.

3 The rationale of root canal therapy is to seal the root canal at the level of the CDJ in order to achieve apical healing. During root canal preparation, care must be taken not to over-instrument the canal by passing through the principal foramen. In dogs and cats with an unmodified apex, the endodontic instruments tend to stop at the end of the root canal (apical terminus) where the small ramifications of the apical delta begin. Subsequently, over-instrumentation is less likely and clinical assessment of working length is easier. Mechanical preparation of the ramifications of the apical delta is impossible and necrotic tissue may remain inside.

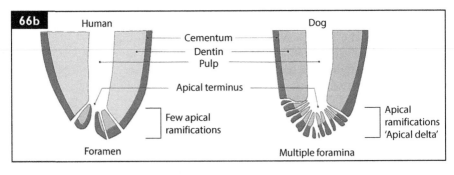

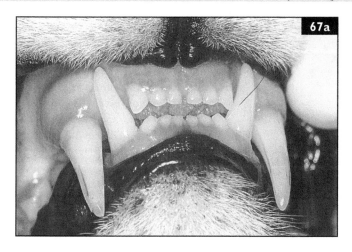

Question 67 Are this cat's mandibular canine teeth normal (**67a**)?

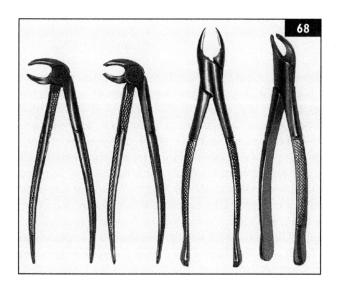

Question 68 Why are extraction forceps less suitable for use in dogs and cats than in humans (**68**)?

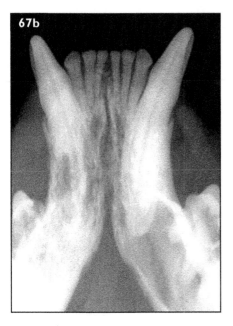

67b

Answer 67 Absence of gingival inflammation, normal sulcus depths, and normal appearance of the crowns leads to a clinical diagnosis of 'normal tooth'. However, the teeth may be very abnormal in their root structure. In the radiograph (**67b**), one canine tooth has a normal crown, but has stage 4c root resorption (see **10**, **12** and **73**). This is defined as resorption causing major loss of substance affecting the root. If the lesion is not exposed to the oral cavity it is believed to be non-painful and does not necessarily require extraction. Coronectomy is the exodontic technique of choice should extraction be elected, as a standard surgical extraction would likely be very traumatic because of the extensive replacement resorption.

Answer 68 Human teeth are relatively robust structures, normally varying only a little in size between patients. Unless they are grossly decayed, human teeth can withstand application of the considerable forces used during forceps extraction. It is necessary for extraction forceps to closely fit the teeth they are applied to, so there are different designs for each size, shape, and position of tooth in the human mouth. Carnivore teeth are relatively thinner, with proportionately longer roots, so are prone to fracture when lateral or crushing forces are applied to them. The teeth also vary considerably in size and form, making it impractical to have an adequate set of forceps for all situations. If forceps are used during extraction of carnivore teeth, the tooth should first be loosened as much as possible using other methods. The instrument jaws are applied as far apically as possible and must fit the tooth well. Pressure is then applied and held repeatedly in an apical then coronal direction, intruding and extruding the tooth into the alveolus to tear periodontal fibers. With single-rooted (reasonably straight) tooth segments, gentle rotational forces can also be applied and held in alternate directions, again tearing periodontal fibers. Use of excessive force is likely to result in tooth or jaw fracture.

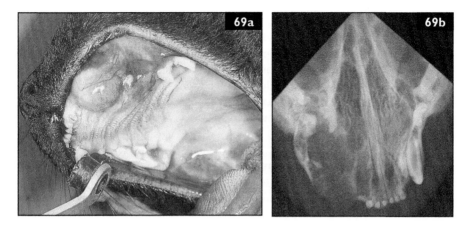

Question 69 This is an oral tumor found in an 18-month-old cat (**69a, b**).
1 What is your tentative radiologic diagnosis?
2 What is known about this tumor type?

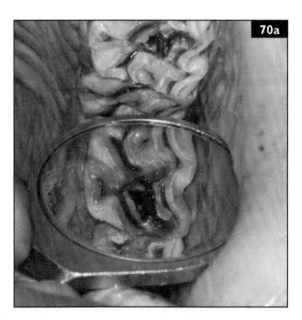

Question 70
1 What lesion of equine teeth is evident here (70a)?
2 At what stage would this lesion become clinically evident, and what would be the presenting signs?

69, 70: Answers

Answer 69

1 This is a typical example of a feline inductive odontogenic tumor.
2 The feline inductive odontogenic tumor, originally described as inductive fibroameloblastoma, is an uncommon tumor type occurring mainly in young cats. It is characterized by ameloblastic epithelial cells arranged around dental pulp-like stroma. The rostral maxilla is the most common site of occurrence. The tumor may be locally invasive, but metastasis has not been recorded.

Answer 70

1 Infundibular caries arises from cemental hypoplasia of the infundibular lakes, which allows the infundibulum to become impacted with food. The food impaction leads to decay of the remaining infundibular cementum and the enamel that encircles the infundibular lakes. There are no infundibula in the mandibular teeth and therefore this condition is confined to the maxilla. Although the disorder can be seen in 80% of horses aged 15 years and over, only a minority of these animals will show clinical signs. In order of frequency, lesions are seen in the first molar, second molar, second premolar, third premolar, fourth premolar and third molar teeth (70b).
2 It is only when the necrosis reaches the pulp cavity that the tooth becomes devitalized, and even then the infection may be contained in some instances. Extension of infection through the apex of the tooth precipitates suppuration in the adjacent tissues, but pathologic fractures of the teeth along a line of weakness between the infundibula accelerate this process. The suppuration in tissues adjacent to the tooth roots is responsible for some cases of secondary maxillary sinusitis.

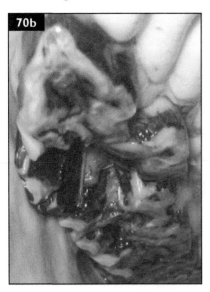
70b

Horses with maxillary periapical abscessation, regardless of mode of origin, are likely to be presented with a facial swelling, possibly with discharging tracts when the second to fourth premolar teeth are diseased and secondary maxillary sinusitis with a putrid nasal discharge when the fourth premolar tooth and first–third molar teeth are involved. In clinical practice, almost all facial swellings which arise rostral to the rostral limit of the facial crest are caused by dental abscessation, and yet very few swellings caudal to this line (i.e. over the maxillary sinuses) themselves arise through periapical infection. Only those patients where displaced fragments of tooth irritate the oral mucosa are likely to show evidence of dysphagia.

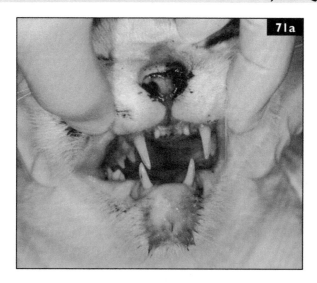

Question 71 A 6-year-old cat was presented for emergency treatment after
being hit-by-car. The mandible is deviated to the right, and the jaws do not
appear to close completely (71a). The
right eye appears mildly exophthalmic
with more sclera visible on the right in
comparison to the left eye, and there
is a perceptible slight increase in ocular retropulsion on the right. A size
#2 digital sensor was used to obtain
initial extraoral dental radiographs of
the TMJ region.

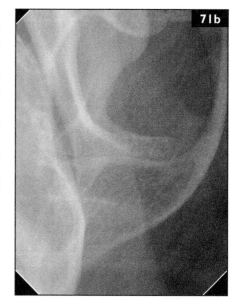

1 What does this radiograph (71b) reveal?
2 Are there other diagnostics tests that are warranted?
3 What treatment is recommended?

Question 72
1 What are biofilms in dental unit waterlines?
2 What are the current recommendations for dental unit waterline quality?
3 What strategies can be implemented to decrease dental unit waterline contamination?

71, 72: Answers

Answer 71

1 This is a luxation of the right condylar process; combined with the mandibular displacement to side of the luxation, pressure of the coronoid process retrobulbar to the right eye is consistent with caudoventral luxation of the right condylar process.

2 When available to the practitioner, computed tomography, either cone-beam or 64-multidetector array, is a superior diagnostic modality compared to traditional skull or extraoral dental radiographs for tri-dimensional assessment of the temporomandibular joint. In this case, computed tomography would be particularly useful in confirming the type of luxation (i.e. rostrodorsal or caudoventral) and identification of fractures of the retroarticular process.

3 In cats, rostrodorsal luxation is the more common injury, and in acute cases, can often be manually reduced using an appropriately sized syringe casing as a fulcrum while simultaneously gently distracting the mandible in a rostral direction (**71c**). For chronic luxations where there is severe masticatory muscle spasm/contracture, caudoventral luxations, or luxations associated with intra-articular fracture, an open/surgical approach (i.e. condylectomy) may be necessary – see **104**. Where there is a perceived likelihood or documented relapse, a tape muzzle, elastomeric chains (**71d**), or traditional maxillomandibular fixation, may be indicated to minimize movement for 2–4 weeks. If traditional maxillomandibular fixation is required, placement of a feeding tube is recommended to ensure delivery of medication and adequate nutrition. The flexible/corrugated section of a drinking straw, preferably a clear straw, to allow efficient penetration of the curing light, is cut to fit, fenestrated, and is placed over the canine teeth as a mold for the light-cured flowable composite material (**71e**). Use of a mold-type technique for fixation of the canine teeth promotes a stronger bond between the teeth, which is favorable while the fixation is needed, but in turn does make it

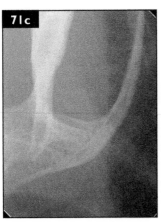

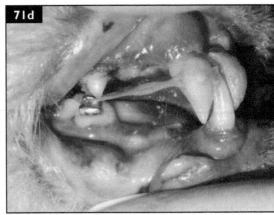

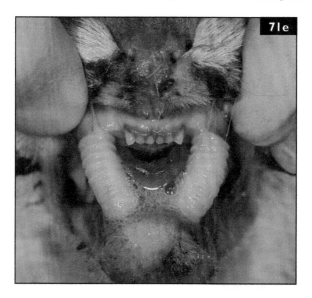

more difficult to remove without traumatizing the underlying teeth. Selecting a shade of composite that differs significantly in color from that of the normal teeth color, and applying the light-cured bonding agent to only the gingival one-third to one-half of the crown, facilitates safe removal of the composite without iatrogenic tooth trauma.

Answer 72

1 Biofilms are well-organized communities of microcolonies that develop on moist surfaces such as dental unit waterlines. Untreated dental unit waterlines may have levels of bacteria in the water exceeding 200,000 colony-forming unit (CFU)/mL in as little as 5 days after installation. The narrow-/small-bore diameter and low-flow environment of dental unit waterlines is an excellent breeding ground for bacteria, fungi, and protozoans that coat the inner lining of the tubing. Stagnant water in the narrow lumen of the tubing promotes precipitation of water molecules that allow for the adherence of phenotype-changing bacteria, which then produce exopolysaccharides that form a protective slime layer around the organisms, shielding them from antibiotics and disinfectants. As water flows through the narrow-diameter tubing, bacteria are shed from the inner surface of the tubing into the patient's mouth.

2 Although infection from dental unit waterline contamination appears to be rare in people, and virtually undocumented in veterinary patients, logically, immunocompromised or geriatric patients may be placed at unnecessary risk for developing infections if exposed to contaminated water, and providing contaminated water to patients is against standard infection protocols. According to

71, 72: Answers

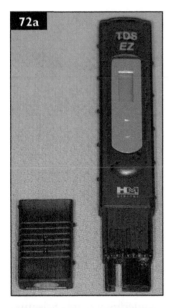

72a

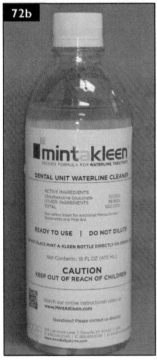

72b

the American Dental Association guidelines that have been in place since 1994, dental unit water should meet or exceed the quality of standard safe normal drinking water and contain <500 CFU/mL of heterotrophic bacteria. Distilled water should be used as the water of choice as a non-sterile coolant/irrigant, and this can help to meet water quality specifications, but does not influence the development of biofilms in water-lines, or affect the purity of the water reaching the patient if biofilms are present in the water-lines. The purity of the distilled water used in dental systems should also be periodically moni-tored with a water tester that measures parts per million (ppm); hand-held monitors are both inex-pensive and readily available (72a).

3 Historically, flushing of the waterlines at the beginning of the work day or the use of dis-tilled water containing <500 CFU/mL alone were believed to be sufficient methods for reducing microbial load. Both methodologies, however, have since been disproven as effective strategies for doing so, and primary treatment/inactivation of the biofilm with a germicide (72b) is still neces-sary. One such product on the market is a liquid 0.12% chlorhexidine gluconate-based product (Mint-A-Kleen®, Anodia Systems), which is used to flush through the lines on a weekly basis, whereas other products, such as CitriSil Blue™ (Sterisil), are stabilized silver tablets that are added to the water supply and are used as a continuous disin-fectant with no appreciable taste difference in the water and just a bluish tinge added to the color of the water. Although the majority of modern power scalers, high-speed handpieces, and water syringes have anti-retraction valves to prevent backflow of oral fluids from the patient, flushing of dental unit waterlines for 20–30 seconds between patients to physically flush the lines is still recommended to discharge any contaminants that may have been retracted.

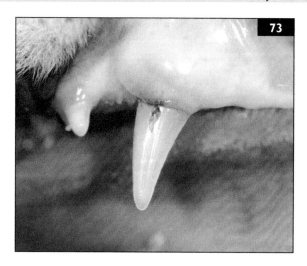

Question 73 Teeth like this (73) are likely to be painful, and something must be done for these cats (see also case 94). Affected teeth should be extracted (see 12 and 55), but is it essential to remove the entire tooth?

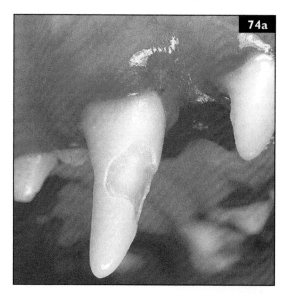

Question 74 What technique could be used to improve the adhesion of composite resin restorative material to the tooth (74a)?

73, 74: Answers

Answer 73 As noted in **67**, teeth with tooth resorption affecting the root but with an intact crown and gingival margin are usually asymptomatic, and deliberate retention of roots in selected cases ('coronectomy') can lead to a pain-free mouth and healthy gingiva over the extraction wound. Coronectomy is a justifiable option if: (1) There is no stomatitis in the area immediately adjacent to the tooth. (2) There is no periodontitis present. (3) There is no radiographic or clinical evidence of endodontic or periapical disease affecting that tooth. If these three criteria are met, the crown and enough root may be removed so that the resorbing root is below the level of remaining bone, and the gingival tissues are sutured over the resorbing root.

Answer 74 Adhesion of dental materials can be by mechanical interlock and by achieving micromechanical retention and sealing. Enamel and dentin are different structures and require different treatment to achieve bonding. Enamel should be etched with a 30–40% phosphoric acid gel (**74b**). Dentin may be etched with phosphoric acid as well, but requires a shorter application time. With the classic total-etch technique, both the enamel and dentin are etched with phosphoric acid. Enamel may require etching times up to 30 seconds. Dentin etching is performed to remove the so-called 'smear layer' and open up the dentinal tubules, allowing improved penetration of the restorative material. Compared to enamel etching, dentin etching requires a shorter time, 15 seconds, and is a more technique-sensitive process than enamel etching. Over-etching, over-drying or etching of dentin prior to use of self-etch adhesive systems may increase postoperative sensitivity, destroy the integrity of the dentinal tubules, and weaken the bond strength. Newer single-bottle self-etch adhesive systems are all-inclusive, combining the process of etching, priming, and bonding dentin. These self-etch systems use acidic monomers to prime and etch dentin, and compared to total-etched dentin, where the smear layer is removed, self-etching systems incorporate the smear layer into a hybrid layer. Water is used as a solvent with self-etch systems therefore over-drying dentin is usually

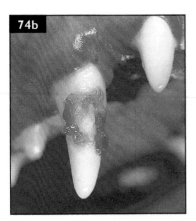

less of a concern. When using the total-etch technique, the next step typically is to apply a bonding agent. The aim of modern bonding agents is to create a link between enamel and dentin (which contain water) and the composite resins which are hydrophobic. By doing so, the bonding strength between the restorative material and the tooth is increased. After application and curing of the bonding agent, the composite resin is applied to the tooth. The composite resin is then placed incrementally in 2–3 mm layers to build up the restoration. This composite resin bonds to the previously applied filled restorative material.

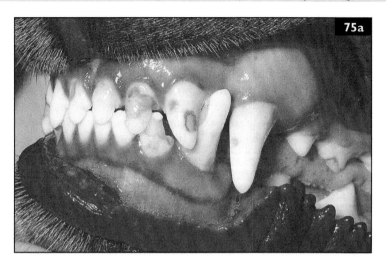

Question 75

1 In the dog shown (75a), what is your diagnosis, and which dental hard tissue is disturbed?
2 How can the different phases in the development of this dental hard tissue be distinguished and their disturbances explained?

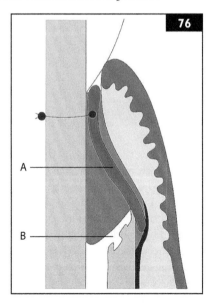

Question 76 What is this technique called (76) and what are the major principles involved?

75, 76: Answers

Answer 75

1 Enamel hypoplasia; the enamel is disturbed.

2 The development of enamel occurs in two phases: (1) the enamel matrix formation stage, and (2) the maturation phase during which the mineralization of the enamel takes place. Disturbances during amelogenesis can cause hypoplasia, hypomineralization, or a combination of both. These conditions may be caused by systemic, local, or hereditary factors and can affect both dentitions.

Enamel hypoplasia is defined as an incomplete or defective formation of the organic enamel component. In cases of enamel hypoplasia, there exists a deficiency in the thickness of the enamel: the defects in the enamel can be limited to a circumscribed area or be recognized as a single narrow zone of smooth or pitted hypoplasia.

If maturation is lacking or incomplete, enamel hypomineralization will develop (**75b**). The mineral content of the enamel is deficient and therefore the enamel persists as a soft enamel matrix. Shortly after eruption the hypomin-

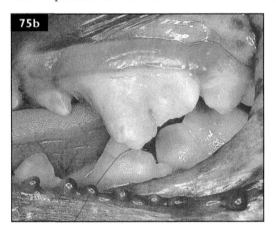

eralized teeth show normal shape, but the surfaces appear dull. Enamel is opaque but the soft enamel matrix will be discolored by extrinsic factors (yellow–brownish). In cases of hypomineralization, the quality of the enamel is abnormal. The lower the mineral content of the enamel, the faster will discoloration be seen and the faster the soft and brittle enamel will peel off.

Answer 76 The barrier (A) over the infrabony defect (B) signifies guided tissue regeneration surgery. The defect must regenerate from cell populations with bone and periodontal ligament characteristics. The barrier excludes gingival connective tissue and oral epithelium which proliferates more rapidly and would otherwise fill a significant portion of the defect. Thus, guided tissue regeneration often allows regrowth of bone and periodontal ligament where it had formerly been lost due to periodontitis. Successfully treated teeth may have stronger support and may have improved long-term survival rates because deep active infrabony pockets are not as likely to recur. Resorbable barriers are most commonly used.

If bone regeneration is desired, a bone graft or substitute is used in addition to the barrier. Growth factors have been used experimentally and the results have been encouraging.

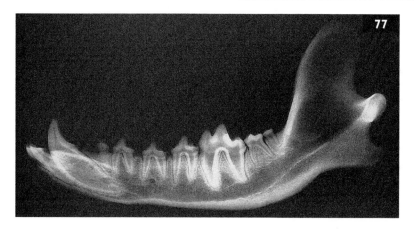

Question 77 The bony portion of the jaw in which the dental roots are located is called the alveolar process (77).
1 What is the structure and composition of the alveolar bone?
2 What is its relationship with the teeth?
3 What is the lamina dura?

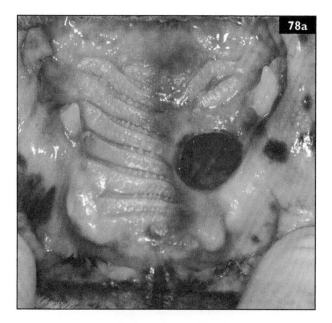

Question 78 Radiation treatment for a squamous cell carcinoma resulted in this palatal defect (78a). What salvage procedure may be indicated in these cases?

Answer 77

1 The alveolar process consists of an outer bony plate of varying thickness and covered by periosteum (the cortical bone), an inner, heavily perforated bony lamella (the alveolar bone proper or cribriform plate), and cancellous bone between the two bony plates and between the alveoli of adjacent teeth. The outer cortical plate is continuous with the inner plate (cribriform plate) at the orifice of the alveolus and this part of the alveolar process is called the alveolar margin. The structure of the cortical plates and of the cancellous bone is similar to that of other bones. The cortical plate of the mandible is thicker than that of the maxilla. The dry weight of alveolar bone is made of about 70% inorganic material (calcium phosphate crystals of the hydroxyapatite type and amorphous calcium phosphate) and 30% organic material (90% collagen).

2 The alveolar margin is located at about 1 mm below the neck of the tooth. The alveolar bone is a tooth-dependent structure, developing with the eruption of the tooth and resorbing after its loss. The cribriform plate is attached to the trabeculae of the cancellous bone. The multiple foramina of this inner plate correspond to the Volkmann canals and connect the periodontal ligament to the bone marrow spaces. Blood and lymph vessels as well as nerves pass through these openings. The surface of the alveolar bone proper adjacent to the periodontal ligament is made of multiple layers of bone parallel to the surface of the alveolar wall, which are penetrated by bundles of Sharpey's fibers embedded almost perpendicular to the surface.

3 On a radiograph, the cribriform plate appears as a radiopaque line distinct from the cancellous bone, which is called the lamina dura. This denser line appears because of an overlapping effect and not because it is more mineralized that the surrounding bone.

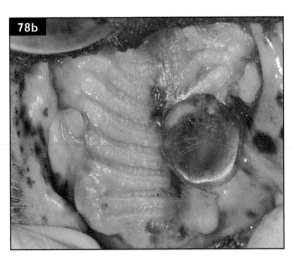

78b

Answer 78 A removable palatal obturator, either acrylic retained by the cheek teeth or a simple vinyl polysiloxane plug (**78b**), can be placed over the defect and adjacent tissue before eating and removed after eating. The obturator serves to shunt food from the turbinates while eating or drinking.

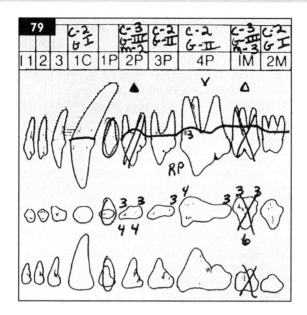

Question 79 Interpret the chart (79), and describe the periodontal status of the teeth shown.

Question 80 Studies have shown that more than 50% of practicing human dentists experience work-related musculoskeletal pain that starts as early as their third year of dental school. These pain disorders begin as microtrauma to the musculoskeletal system as a result of poor operator posture, positioning, and operatory layout. The tissue damage that occurs is normally repaired by the body during periods of rest, but when there is insufficient rest, the tissue damage accumulates in the form of cumulative trauma disorders (CTD). Although similar pain disorder prevalence studies for the practicing veterinary dentist do not exist, with many veterinary dental work stations being afterthought additions to the veterinary clinic, the working conditions and knowledge about CTD by veterinary personnel are likely to be inadequate.
1 What are the most common CTD in dentistry?
2 What are important ergonomic considerations when selecting an operator stool, dental loupes and lighting systems?

Question 81 When repairing mandibular and maxillary fractures in the dog and cat, how can an adequate airway for anesthesia, good surgical exposure, and the opportunity to check the occlusion intraoperatively be achieved?

Answer 79 Only abnormalities are noted. Interpretation of the symbols and letter codes on the diagnostic chart illustrated describing the periodontal status of this left maxilla would be as follows: (1) Canine tooth: calculus index 2, gingival index 1, probing depths within normal limits. (2) First premolar tooth: missing. (3) Second premolar tooth: calculus index 3, gingival index 3, stage of mobility 2, stage 3 furcation lesion, and probing depth of 3 mm buccally and 4 mm palatally with 2 mm gingival recession over the furcation area. (4) Third premolar tooth: calculus index 2, gingival index 2, 3 mm probing depth at the distal/buccal aspect. (5) Fourth premolar tooth: calculus index 2, gingival index 2, 3 mm gingival recession over the mesiobuccal root with 4 mm probing depth, a stage 1 furcation lesion, and 2 mm gingival recession over the distal root with 3 mm probing depth at the distal aspect. (6) First molar tooth: calculus index 3, gingival index 2, stage of mobility 3, 4 mm gingival recession buccally and stage 3 furcation lesion, probing depth of 3 mm buccally and 6 mm at the palatal root. (7) Second molar tooth: calculus index 2, gingival index 1, and probing depths within normal limits. These are only a sampling of the symbols and letter abbreviations that can be used to denote dental changes. The reader is referred to additional references for further information on charting.

In summary, these findings are consistent with:

Stage 1 periodontal disease: canine, third premolar and second molar teeth;

Stage 2 periodontal disease: fourth premolar tooth;

Stage 4 periodontal disease: second premolar and first molar teeth.

Stages of periodontal disease (American Veterinary Dental College, 2005)	
Stage	Definition
0	Normal.
1	Gingivitis only without attachment loss – the height and architecture of the alveolar margin are normal.
2	Early periodontitis implies that there is less than 25% of attachment loss. There are early radiologic signs of periodontitis. The loss of periodontal attachment is less than 25% as measured either by probing of the clinical attachment level, or radiographic determination of the distance of the alveolar margin from the cementoenamel junction relative to the length of the root, or there is a stage 1 furcation involvement in multirooted teeth.
3	Moderate periodontitis implies that there is 25–50% of attachment loss as measured either by probing of the clinical attachment level, or radiographic determination of the distance of the alveolar margin from the cementoenamel junction relative to the length of the root, or there is a stage 2 furcation involvement in multirooted teeth.

4   Advanced periodontitis implies that there is more than 50% of attachment loss as measured either by probing of the clinical attachment level, or radiographic determination of the distance of the alveolar margin from the cementoenamel junction relative to the length of the root, or there is a stage 3 furcation involvement in multirooted teeth.

Answer 80

1 Carpal tunnel syndrome, rotator cuff impingement, tension neck syndrome, chronic low-back pain and trapezius myalgia.

2 *Operator stools* (80). The proper seated posture for veterinary dentists should allow for the hips to be higher than the knees to reduce disc pressure/muscle activity in the lower back and preserve the lumbar curve. To achieve this posture, the seat pan of the stool should be tilted slightly downward (5–15°). A saddle-type stool or a wedge-shaped foam cushion can be used with a non-tilted seat pan to achieve a similar effect. Seat pan depths range from 14–18 inches and should support most of the operator's thighs. A backrest for lumbar support, sturdy five-caster base with appropriate casters for the floor type, adjustable armrests to prevent back, neck and shoulder pain, and an optimal cylinder height (ranging between 16–21 inches for short operators and between 21–26 inches for tall operators), are all components that are considered ideal for an ergonomic operator stool.

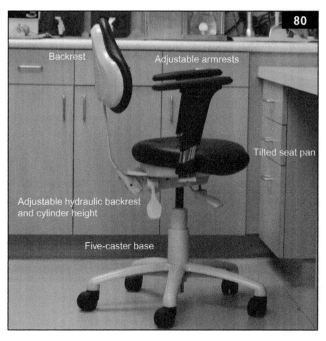

Dental loupes. Two basic types of loupes, through-the-lens (TTL) and flip-ups, are available. Well-designed dental loupes should allow for less than 25° of forward head posture. For the general veterinary dentist a magnification strength of 2.5–3.5× is recommended. The declination angle is a term that refers to the angle that your eyes are inclined downward toward the working area; when selecting loupes, the steepest declination angle should be specified. Positioning the scopes as low as possible with respect to the pupils is also ideal, as it promotes better working posture, and compared to TTL loupes, flip-up scopes typically allow for lower positioning. The distance from the eyes to the working area is known as the working distance, and should be measured in a neutral seated position at the dental treatment table (i.e. 14 inches or less for shorter veterinarians and more than 20 inches for taller veterinarians) where the loupes will be used.

Lighting systems. Overhead lighting, even in combination with the fiberoptic/LED lighting of handpieces, is often inadequate for illumination; spot/task lighting with a headlamp attached to the dental loupe frame or to a separate headband provides an indispensable boost in visual acuity. Task lighting provides line-of-sight lighting, eliminates shadows, and reduces eyes strain. As a general rule when selecting a task light, the intensity of the task light should not be more than 10 times as bright as the ambient lighting (typically 3,000 lux). Weight of the light, spot size, color temperature, and battery life are other features that should be considered when purchasing a task light.

Answer 81 Passing the endotracheal tube through a pharyngotomy incision satisfies all requirements (**81**). The importance of checking the occlusion during surgical repair of mandibular and maxillary fractures cannot be overemphasized. The presence of an oral endotracheal tube makes this impossible. However, intubation with a cuffed endotracheal tube to prevent aspiration is highly recommended during any oral surgery. Care should be taken to use a wire-reinforced endotracheal tube, to

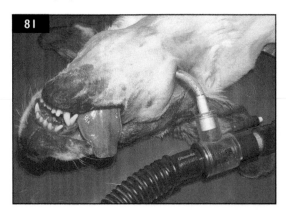

prevent collapse of the tube when bent. An additional advantage of a pharyngotomy is that the same opening may be used postoperatively for a gastroesophageal tube for nutritional support. Contrary to tracheotomy, pharyngotomy is a safe and easy procedure. Alternatively orotracheal intubation can be achieved using a transmylohyoid approach.

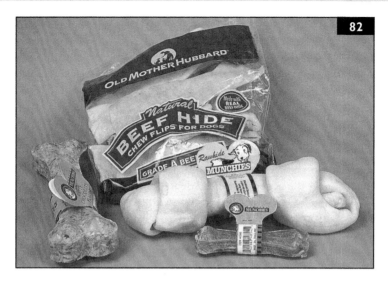

Question 82 Chew treats may be beneficial in maintaining periodontal health (**82**).
1 What benefits can be expected from chew treats?
2 Describe the proposed mechanisms of action.
3 With the plethora of dental products available in the marketplace, are there certain products that are more efficacious than others for retarding plaque and calculus?

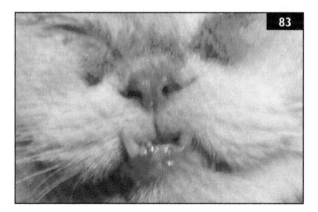

Question 83
1 What common orthodontic problem in purebred cats is seen here (**83**)?
2 What are the treatment options and expected results?
3 What are the dental show standards for cats?

Answer 82

1 Depending on the type of treat, the act of chewing may reduce the accumulation of dental deposits (plaque and calculus) on the tooth surfaces, and a reduction in plaque may reduce gingivitis. Most chew-type treats need to be offered on a daily basis, palatable enough that the dog or cat will accept the treat, and of a consistency that will promote chewing.

2 Specialized dental treats, in addition to being dependent on chewing action, are either intrinsically designed for the mechanical removal of dental deposits, or have a chemical ingredient, typically a polyphosphate, that is incorporated into the treat as an ingredient, or a chemical that is sprayed onto the surface of the treat that reduces the accumulation of dental plaque and/or calculus.

3 The Veterinary Oral Health Council (VOHC) is an organization modelled after the American Dental Association that serves to award products with a Seal of Acceptance that meet a pre-set standard of plaque and calculus retardation in dogs and cats. This process has yielded a consumer-friendly list of products including diets, treats, tooth coatings, water additives, gels, sprays, toothpastes, and toothbrushes that have demonstrated a minimum 20% reduction in plaque and/or calculus compared to a control group in two separate trials. These VOHC-accepted products must also demonstrate safety, must not produce physical damage to the oral tissues, and if a chemical agent is used, the product must meet the federal designation as Generally Regarded As Safe (GRAS).

Answer 83

1 The development of brachycephalic feline breeds has resulted in a wry malocclusion and craniofacial asymmetry often associated with one mandibular canine tooth in an extraoral position when the mouth is closed.

2 Restoration of the dentition to a normal occlusion is extremely difficult. This condition is usually not amenable to orthodontic correction. If orthodontic correction is attempted, fixed dental attachments (i.e. hooks, buttons) are placed on the deviated canine tooth and on one or more anchor teeth. The maxillary fourth premolar and the mandibular first molar teeth are often used as anchor teeth. Elastic traction (i.e. power chain, rubber bands) creates constant force on the canine tooth. Leaving this untreated can result in continued soft-tissue trauma to the upper lip, masticatory impairment, and periodontal complications. Crown reduction and vital pulp therapy, followed by home care, is another option to relieve upper lip trauma and improve masticatory function.

3 Feline show standards are rather non-specific. They usually state that no teeth are to be visible when the mouth is closed. This simple standard does not address occlusion nor disqualification for correction. The American Veterinary Medical Association (AVMA) ethical guidelines are discussed in **183**.

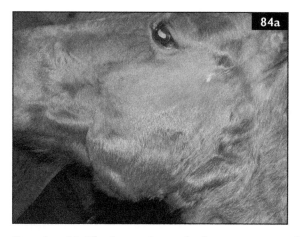
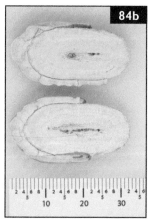

Question 84 The horse shown had a tortuous swelling on the left side of the face (84a). The structure (which has been bisected) was surgically removed from this horse's parotid salivary duct (84b).
1 What is it?
2 What is the pathogenesis of this condition?

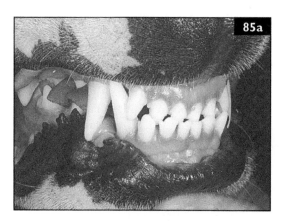

Question 85
1 Describe three possible etiologies for this malocclusion (85a).
2 Name the two principal means of moving teeth to correct a rostral crossbite, and briefly describe the techniques and risks.
3 Describe the sequelae of no treatment.

84, 85: Answers

Answer 84

1 A sialolith.

2 An ascending foreign body, in this case a grass awn, is usually the cause of a single sialolith within a salivary duct. The sialolith consists of concentric layers of mostly calcium phosphate crystals around the organic nucleus. They are usually elongated in shape. In the dog and cat, dystrophic calcification of inspissated saliva in salivary mucoceles may also result in sialolith formation; in these cases, multiple small sialoliths may be present. A single, large sialolith located in a salivary duct may give rise to some retention of saliva but is generally believed not to cause a salivary mucocele. Sialoliths should be removed intraorally. The mucosa and parotid duct is incised over the sialolith and the sialolith delivered into the mouth. The incision is left to heal by second intention.

Answer 85

1 (1) Persistent deciduous incisor teeth can result in palatal or lingual displacement of the permanent incisor teeth. Persistent deciduous teeth in humans are believed to be of genetic origin in that the permanent tooth bud is displaced away from the deciduous precursor and cannot cause a resorptive action upon the deciduous root. (2) Discrepancy in jaw length (relative maxillary brachygnathia, class III malocclusion or mandibular mesiocclusion) alters the normal occlusal relationship of the incisor teeth. (3) Trauma to the maxilla or mandible of a neonate or juvenile can result in an acquired rostral crossbite. Displacement of the permanent incisor tooth bud results in an abnormal path of eruption.

2 The two means of movement are mechanical or surgical. Mechanical movement requires placement of an orthodontic appliance (85b). Commonly used appliances are arch wires and various screw-type expansion devices. The risks include periodontal trauma, root resorption, failure to move, and relapse. Sur-

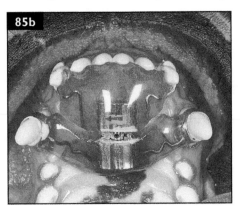

85b

gical movement involves resection of periodontal hard and soft tissues and repositioning of the tooth/teeth. Risks include perioperative extraction and postoperative endodontic complications; surgical movement therefore cannot be recommended.

3 Rostral crossbite rarely requires correction for the health and welfare of the patient. There is no masticatory interference or soft-tissue trauma and rarely any periodontal involvement.

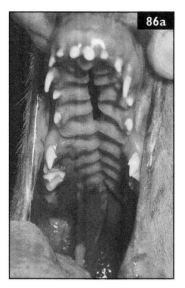
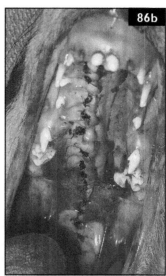

Question 86 This is a congenital cleft hard palate with an associated midline soft-palatal defect in a 4-month-old Collie presented because of chronic, bilateral nasal discharge (**86a, b**). Several guidelines have been recommended in the surgical management of congenital cleft hard- and soft-palatal defects. What are these guidelines and what surgical technique can be utilized in the successful management of congenital cleft hard- and soft-palatal defects?

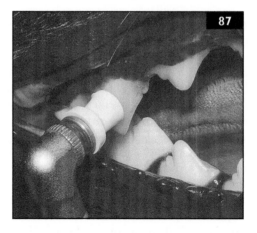

Question 87 What procedure is being performed and what is the rationale for doing so (**87**)?

Answer 86 The following guidelines have been recommended in the surgical management of palatal defects: (1) The covering flaps should be larger than the defect they will cover. (2) The vascular supply to the flap should be preserved. (3) Suture lines should be arranged whenever possible to lie over connective tissue rather than over the defect. (4) Tissues should be handled gently and relatively large bites of tissue should be taken to minimize tension and minimize interference with the blood supply at the edges of the wound. (5) The use of electrocoagulation for hemorrhage control should be avoided. (6) Tissues should be sutured to appose edges that do not have an intact epithelial surface. (7) A two-layer closure should be utilized whenever possible.

The surgical techniques that utilize the guidelines listed above are the overlapping flap technique for the repair of hard-palatal defects and the two-layer closure of the soft-palatal congenital defect. The overlapping flap technique is preferred by most surgeons because there is less tension on the suture line, the suture line is not located directly over the defect, and the area of opposing connective tissue is larger which results in a stronger scar. The overlapping flap technique is performed by creating two mucoperiosteal flaps. One flap is hinged at the end of the palatal defect and is turned beneath the other flap. Horizontal mattress sutures of synthetic absorbable suture material are utilized to maintain the connective tissue surfaces of both flaps in apposition. The midline soft-palatal defect is corrected by making an incision along the medial margin of the soft palate on each side and blunt separating the palatal tissue to form a dorsal and ventral flap on each side with scissors. The two dorsal flaps are sutured in a simple-interrupted pattern while the two ventral flaps are sutured.

Answer 87 The tooth is being polished using the standard cup-and-pumice technique. Scaling may leave the tooth surfaces roughened, making it easier for the plaque to adhere. It is therefore common practice to make the dental surfaces as smooth as possible. However, the long-term beneficial effect of polishing would appear to be minimal. In addition, iatrogenic loss of enamel and cementum may occur as a result of overzealous polishing. Therefore 'selective polishing' is recommended, which consists of polishing the surfaces with palpable irregularities.

Polishing the teeth can be performed using a low-speed handpiece, a rubber prophylaxis cup and pumice. The rubber cup is filled with a slurry of a mildly abrasive prophylaxis paste or pumice polish. The slow-speed unit may be powered by compressed air or an electric motor. It should be rotated at less than 3,000 rpm, using only enough pressure to slightly flare the edge of the cup. Using too fast a rotation speed, too little paste, or polishing for too long a time on one tooth can all generate heat which can injure the pulp. A disposable, oscillating prophylaxis angle offers the advantage of avoiding entanglement of fur.

Question 88 This dog had a history of a shifting limb lameness. In addition to findings noted in the oral cavity (**88**), the clinical and laboratory examination revealed lethargy, mild peripheral lymphadenopathy, mild fever, and confirmed proteinuria with no other abnormalities on a complete urinalysis. The results of a complete blood count and biochemical profile were within normal limits.

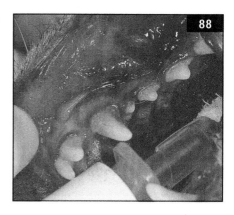

1 This patient should be evaluated for which autoimmune disease?

2 Which diagnostic tests are indicated to evaluate for autoimmune disease?

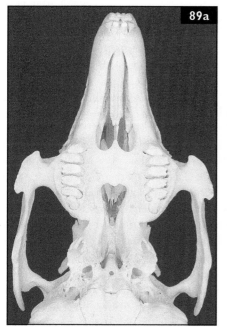

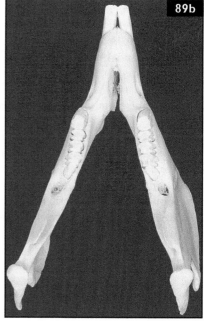

Question 89

1 State the dental formula and characteristic dental features of the domestic rabbit (**89a, b**).

2 How does the dentition of lagomorphs differ from that of rodents?

Answer 88

1 Systemic lupus erythematosus (SLE) is an autoimmune disease that affects multiple organ systems. Polyarthritis and/or polymyositis are common in SLE and may result in a stiff gait or a shifting limb lameness. Cutaneous lesions are common and include lesions affecting the body, limbs, head, mucocutaneous junctions, and oral cavity. Major signs of SLE include non-erosive polyarthritis, polymyositis, bullous dermatitis, proteinuria, and immune-mediated hemolytic anemia and/or thrombocytopenia and/or leukopenia. Minor signs include oral ulceration, pleuritis, myocarditis, pericarditis, peripheral lymphadenopathy, fever of unknown origin, dementia, and seizures.

2 The diagnosis of SLE is based on a combination of clinical signs and laboratory tests. The extent of the diagnostic evaluation is determined by the clinical signs and initial laboratory database. Serologic tests used to support a diagnosis of SLE include an indirect fluorescent antinuclear antibody test (ANA test) and lupus erythematosus cell test (LE cell test). The diagnosis of SLE is usually made when two major signs are present with a positive serologic test. A probable diagnosis is made when one major sign and a positive serologic test are present or two major signs with negative serologic tests. When evaluating the results of ANA and LE cell tests the laboratory should be consulted to determine the significance of the ANA titers and the possibilities for false-positive and false-negative results.

Answer 89

1 The dental formula of lagomorphs is: $I\frac{2}{1}:C\frac{0}{0}:P\frac{3}{2}:M\frac{3}{3}=28$

Rabbits have a heterodont, diphyodont dentition with all teeth being elodont (aradicular hypsodont): elodont teeth grow throughout life and never develop anatomic roots. Although diphyodont, the deciduous teeth are not functional and are exfoliated shortly before or after birth. The incisor teeth are separated from the premolar teeth and molar teeth by a wide interdental space, often incorrectly referred to as 'diastema', without canine teeth. There is a pair of small maxillary second incisor teeth, the 'peg teeth', behind the large first incisor teeth. All incisor teeth have a complete covering of enamel.

2 The main taxonomic difference is the presence of the maxillary second incisor teeth in lagomorphs, while rodents have only a single pair. Another difference is that lagomorphs are diphyodont while rodents are considered monophyodont. Rabbits have unpigmented enamel while most rodents have yellow–orange incisor tooth enamel. Rabbits have a full elodont dentition while in most rodents only the incisor teeth are continuously growing. The relative widths of the mandible and maxilla, and the range of movement of the temporomandibular joint, also form important differences.

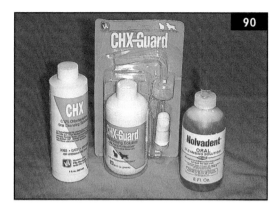

Question 90 Oral antiseptic rinses or gels can be a useful adjunct to mechanical plaque removal (90).
1 List two properties of an oral antiseptic solution that determine its expected effect in the oral cavity.
2 Which is the most proven oral antiseptic solution to date?
3 What formulation and what concentration are generally recommended?
4 What is the main disadvantage of this antiseptic?
5 List two clinical situations where an antiseptic rinse or gel is indicated. Outline the rationale for this recommendation.

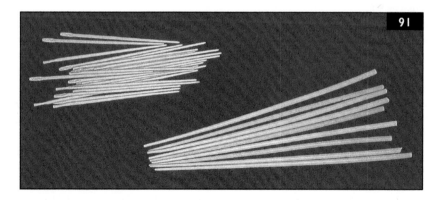

Question 91 Shown here are various sizes of gutta-percha points (91).
1 What is gutta-percha?
2 For what purpose is it used in veterinary dentistry, and what are its main advantages?
3 Are there other dental uses for gutta-percha?

Answer 90

1 Antibacterial spectrum of the antiseptic, and substantivity. Substantivity implies that the adherence of the antiseptic to the oral tissues should be greater or more extended than would occur following simple mechanical deposition.

2 Chlorhexidine.

3 Chlorhexidine gluconate is generally preferred to chlorhexidine diacetate. A 0.12% concentration is widely used in human dentistry, although it has been shown in wound-healing experiments that a 0.05% solution may be preferable because chlorhexidine is less cytotoxic at this concentration. For the same reason, alcohol-free solutions are preferred.

4 The main disadvantage of chlorhexidine is that it may stain the teeth. Moreover, it is inactivated by the presence of organic material. For best results, chlorhexidine should be used together with tooth brushing which physically removes the plaque and reduces tooth staining.

5 Oral antiseptic rinse or gel is used to augment the effect of mechanical plaque removal. It can also be used on its own if mechanical plaque removal is not possible, e.g. due to postoperative pain, but where plaque control is required to allow resolution of inflammation. Two clinical situations where oral antiseptic rinse or gel, preferably in addition to mechanical plaque removal, is very useful are: (1) dogs with contact mucositis and mucosal ulceration; and (2) following gingivectomy and gingivoplasty for gingival enlargement in dogs. Every attempt should be made to institute daily plaque removal by mechanical means as soon as the animal will allow it.

Answer 91

1 Gutta-percha is an inert, flexible material harvested from the maser wood tree and is more commonly used in the softened b-form, which is more flexible and less brittle than the natural a-form. Distributed to the clinician in the b-form, the material transforms to the less flexible and more brittle a-form as its shelf-life expires. Today, most gutta-percha used is actually gutta-bullata, which is harvested from a different species of tree. It has better properties and is more readily available. Gutta-percha points, as both products are commonly called, are only 15–22% gutta-percha. Gutta-percha points consist of 56–79% zinc oxide, the remainder of the material comprising metal sulfides, wax, and resins. Standardized (ISO) gutta-percha points, like absorbent points, are supplied in sizes 15 to 120, and in lengths of 30 mm and 55 mm to correspond to standardized file sizes.

2 Gutta-percha is the most popular endodontic core-filling material used. It is non-irritating to the periapical tissues. Gutta-percha is highly compactable and adapts well to the shape of the prepared root canal by lateral and vertical condensation. It is physicochemically stable and does not shrink.

3 Gutta-percha is radiopaque and can be used as a marker in draining tracts. It also serves conveniently to help clinicians to identify visually the root canal during apicoectomy procedures.

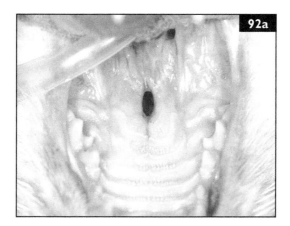

Question 92 This is an intraoral view of a 3-year-old cat that was presented because of a 7 × 12 mm caudal hard-palatal defect of 1-year's duration (**92a**). Several attempts to repair the defect with sliding flaps had been unsuccessful.
1 What are the causes of centrally located hard-palatal defects?
2 Large defects located in the caudal aspect of the hard palate can be frustrating to repair, and postoperative dehiscence is a potential complication. What surgical procedure utilizes flaps based on the blood supply to the hard palate and adjacent soft-tissue structures?
3 What other surgical option is available?

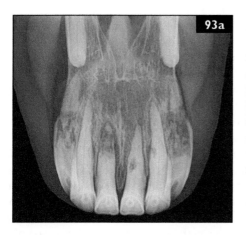
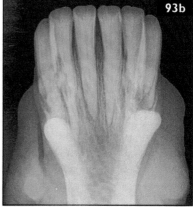

Question 93 This 17-year-old thoroughbred gelding had radiographs obtained of the incisor quadrants (**93a, b**). What is the dental pathology demonstrated on the radiographs and the recommended treatment?

92, 93: Answers

Answer 92

1 Centrally located, acquired hard-palatal defects are mainly of traumatic origin: bite wounds, electrical cord injury, gunshot wounds, foreign body penetration, and pressure necrosis from a foreign body wedged between the two sides of the maxillary dental arcade.

2 The split palatal U-flap can be utilized to repair large caudal hard-palatal defects. In this technique a large mucoperiosteal U-flap is created rostral to the defect and then split along the midline. Each side of the U-flap is gently elevated, taking care not to damage the major palatine arteries as they exit through the major palatine foramina approximately 5–10 mm palatal to the maxillary fourth premolar teeth. Following débridement of the edges of the palatal defect, the

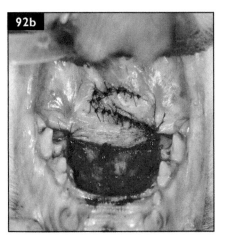

first half of the U-flap is rotated into the palatal defect and sutured in place with synthetic absorbable suture material. The second half of the U-flap is then rotated rostral to the first half of the U-flap and sutured to the edge of the first flap. The rostral aspect of the palate from which the U-flap is harvested is devoid of a mucoperiosteal covering. This exposed bone at the donor site is left to heal by second intention and generally will epithelialize within 1–2 months (92b).

3 Surgical repair using auricular cartilage is another surgical option.

Answer 93 There is resorption of the incisor teeth of this horse. This condition has been described as equine odontoclastic resorption and hypercementosis (EOTRH). Hypercementosis was hypothesized as a reparative process in advanced cases. This case does not have hypercementosis. Tooth resorption in other species has been classified into seven types and is considered a radiologic diagnosis. Tooth resorption can be secondary to other dental pathology and certain types of resorption are idiopathic. The resorptive lesions are described in five stages according to the extent of the tooth structures that are affected.

This case demonstrates a resorptive process where there is a widening of the periodontal ligament with loss of both tooth structure and adjacent alveolar bone. The pulp chamber of the majority of the teeth is involved in the resorptive process, indicating that the vitality of the teeth is compromised. Extraction of the non-vital teeth is the current treatment of choice. Tooth resorption is considered a progressive condition, and teeth with resorptive lesions that are radiographically considered vital are rechecked yearly and radiographs obtained.

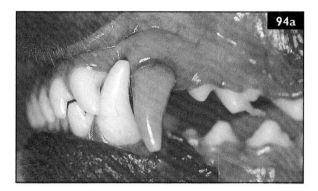

Question 94 Discolorations of teeth can be classified as generalized, local, or pseudodiscolorations.
1 Which type can be seen here (94a), and what are the possible causes?
2 Is treatment necessary and, if performed, will the discoloration disappear?

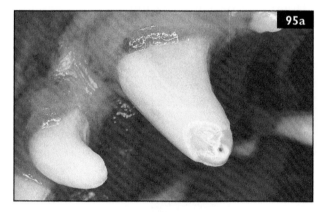

Question 95 In designing a crown for this fractured tooth (95a):
1 Where should the margins be placed?
2 What type of margins could be used, and what are the advantages and disadvantages of each?
3 What is the minimum clinical crown height requirement for placement of a crown?
4 What is the optimal convergence angle for the crown preparation?

Question 96 Conventional endodontic therapy concentrates on the cleaning, shaping, and sealing of the root canal system.
1 What instruments have traditionally been used to shape the apical stop?
2 How do 60-mm veterinary-length root canal instruments differ from ISO-instruments?

Answer 94

1 The list below summarizes the causes of dental discoloration. The case in question is a local discoloration, probably of endodontic–traumatic origin. Hemorrhage or necrosis of the pulp causes lysis of the erythrocytes. The hemoglobin breaks down into pigments which penetrate the dentinal tubules and are responsible for the different discolorations. The color of the crown may vary from pink–red to blue–gray or dark gray. In the case of a minor hemorrhage, the pulp may survive, blood pigments may be resorbed and the discoloration may be transient. In most cases, however, discoloration of the entire crown, as in this case (**94a**), indicates pulp necrosis. Another possible cause of crown discoloration is acute pulpitis of hematogenous origin. A localized pink–red area on the crown may be indicative of vital pulp with internal resorption, the vascular resorbing tissue being visible through the enamel ('pink spot of Mummery' – **94b**, arrowed).

Generalized discolorations: (1) Genetic: amelogenesis imperfecta; dentinogenesis imperfecta; odontodysplasia. (2) Metabolic disturbance (prolonged): enamel hypoplasia; enamel hypomineralization. (3) Ageing: enamel infarction; attrition/abrasion. (4) Iatrogenic: tetracyclines; fluorosis.

Local discolorations: (1) Genetic: odontodysplasia. (2) Metabolic disturbance (short period): enamel hypoplasia; enamel hypomineralization. (3) Ageing: enamel infarction; attrition/abrasion. (4) Trauma/endodontic: pre-eruptive: mechanical/chemical trauma; periapical pathology deciduous tooth; post-eruptive: pulp hemorrhage; pulp necrosis; internal resorption. (5) Dental caries. (6) Iatrogenic: endodontic and restorative materials.

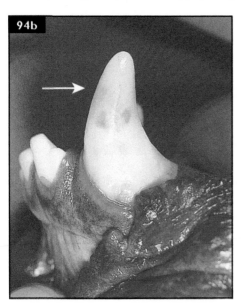

Pseudodiscolorations: (1) Dental plaque and calculus. (2) Agents in food.

2 Radiographic examination and pulp-vitality testing (if available) are indicated and endodontic treatment is most often the treatment of choice. It is important to note that discoloration may persist following endodontic treatment.

Answer 95

1 The crown margins in veterinary patients should be located supragingivally (1–2 mm coronal to the gingival margin). Supragingivally located crown margins are more accessible for plaque control, and are typically associated with less gingival inflammation, less alveolar bone loss, and less gingival recession. Restoration margins cannot be perfectly contoured to the tooth, and any subgingival incongruities, even microscopic defects, will be a focus for plaque retention and will increase gingivitis, gingival recession, and will ultimately compromise the biologic width of the tooth's attachment. The gains in retention and resistance form with a subgingival preparation are negligible, and should not be considered as a reason to create a subgingival preparation. If the crown margin must be placed subgingivally, the chances of doing harm to the periodontium are minimized by creating a well-adapted margin and with implementation of good oral hygiene.

2 There are three general types of margins: (1) A feathered (or knife-edge) margin is where the margin is created by gently sloping the margin coronally (**95b, A**). Often, the actual end point of the margin is not obvious and must be indicated to the laboratory. This margin has the advantages of minimal tooth loss and ease of preparation. (2) A shoulder margin (**95b, B**) is where a definite ledge is created in the prepared tooth. The disadvantage of this margin is the increased amount of tooth loss. It is required for a porcelain crown. A variation of this technique is to add a bevel to the shoulder (**95b, C**). This is indicated for preparations with extremely short walls and can also be used for porcelain-fused-to-metal crowns. (3) A chamfer (**95b, D**) is a hybrid between the feathered margin at one extreme and a shoulder margin at the other. This is generally regarded as the finish line of choice for metal crowns.

3 The veterinary dental literature has propagated the recommendation that 5–8 mm of clinical crown is required for adequate resistance and retention form of a crown. A recently published review of the literature revealed only low-grade evidence to support this recommendation. Furthermore, because of the broad

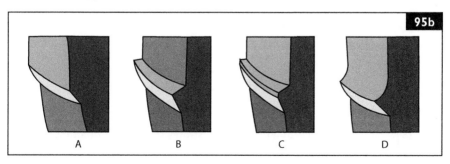

95b

range in clinical tooth size and shape of animal teeth, an exact millimeter recommendation for clinical crown height is unattainable.

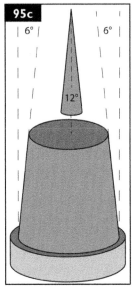

4 The crown form should be created so that there are no overhangs and an optimal 12° convergence angle (taper of 6° on each surface) exists to allow the prosthetic crown to fit properly and have optimal retention (95c). The goal of axial wall reduction in crown preparation is to achieve parallelism to maximize retention and resistance form, and to achieve this with as low a convergence angle as possible. Clinically, the ideal convergence angle (12°) is rarely if at all possible to achieve, and a recent study has shown that convergence angles of greater than 12° can be considered as acceptable, and that the greater the crown height available the less important it is to adhere to the ideal convergence angle. That said, other factors play a role in the success of a crown such as the type of cement used, whether the inner surface of the crown is sand blasted, and if internal parallel grooves are used in the preparation.

Answer 96

1 The apical extent of the root canal is shaped using hand instruments such as K-files, Hedström files, or K-reamers. ISO-standard files and reamers have a diameter of $(1/100 \times \text{ISO-number})$ mm at their tip, increasing in diameter by 0.32 mm along the 16 mm working end. Standardized paper and gutta-percha points are produced with the same taper.

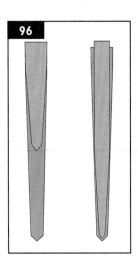

2 Veterinary-length (60 mm) root canal files and reamers have a working end which is about twice as long as the ISO-size equivalent file, with a reduced taper. In order to prepare the apical root canal for placement of standard-sized gutta-percha points it is necessary to use a 'step-back technique' when using 60 mm files. This involves preparing the apex to the master file size required, then continuing preparation with sequentially larger-size files which are worked to within 1 or 2 mm of the depth reached by the previously used file. The diagram (96) illustrates the poor fit of an ISO-standard gutta-percha point in a root canal prepared with a long taper file.

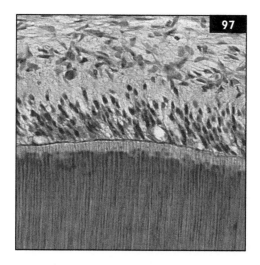

Question 97 The bulk of most mature teeth is composed of dentin (**97**).
1 What are the main components of dentin?
2 What are primary, secondary and tertiary dentin?
3 How is dentin formed?

Question 98 What are important consider-ations and guidelines when obtaining a biopsy of a suspected oral tumor (**98**)?

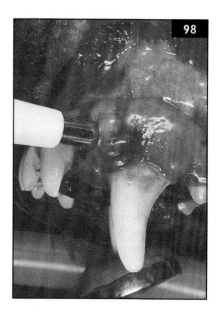

103

Answer 97

1 Dentin is composed of a mineralized collagenous matrix. The mineral component is principally calcium hydroxyapatite.

2 Three types of dentin are recognized. Dentin formed until the external form of the tooth is completed and the tooth erupts, is known as primary dentin. Secondary dentin is the result of the continuing deposition of dentin by the odontoblasts, albeit at a slower rate; this leads to a progressive reduction in the size of the pulp chamber and root canal. Tertiary dentin forms in reaction to noxious stimuli. Tertiary dentin can further be subdivided into reactionary tertiary dentin and reparative tertiary dentin. Reactionary dentinogenesis occurs following stimulation of existing odontoblasts by mild injury to the dentin, such as attrition or slow abrasion. Reparative dentinogenesis follows the differentiation of pulpal progenitor cells into odontoblast-like cells underneath severe injury to the dentin, such as a caries lesion.

3 Dentin is formed by odontoblasts, the cells lining the pulp cavity. These cells lay down a collagenous matrix known as predentin which is then mineralized to form dentin. Throughout life the odontoblasts continue producing secondary dentin, gradually reducing the size of the tooth's pulp cavity. The odontoblasts have long, fine cellular processes, the odontoblastic processes, which extend within the dentinal tubules.

Answer 98 An incisional biopsy is preferred if: (1) One is uncertain whether the lesion is neoplastic. (2) The result of the biopsy might influence the therapeutic plan. (3) The planned therapy is potentially associated with considerable disfigurement and morbidity. (4) The client desires an accurate prognosis.

All of these considerations were valid in the case illustrated (98), which turned out to be a poorly differentiated sarcoma. This case also illustrates the wide variety of histopathologic entities which may clinically present as an *epulis* (see 10). In selected cases of very small tumors on the gingival margin, an excisional biopsy by means of gingivectomy may be indicated where the tumor can easily be excised *in toto*.

In obtaining a biopsy, the following important technical details should be borne in mind: (1) Taking a biopsy must be done as atraumatically as possible, to prevent exfoliation and seeding of neoplastic cells. (2) The site of the biopsy must fall within the boundaries of the tissue to be excised. (3) A representative tissue sample should be obtained and normal tissue should not be included in order to avoid opening previously unopened tissue planes.

The biopsy should be adequately fixed and submitted to a pathologist with experience in oral pathology. The result of the histopathologic examination should be compatible with the clinical findings; if not, the matter should be discussed with the pathologist. If any doubt remains, an additional biopsy may be indicated.

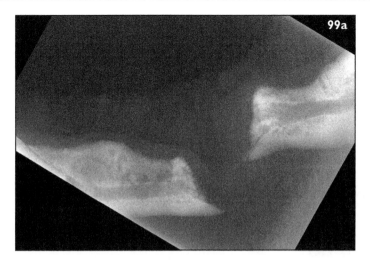

Question 99 This 8-year-old Shih Tzu sustained a mandibular fracture 2 years ago and several attempts at repair have been unsuccessful (**99a**).
1 Describe the radiologic findings.
2 What type of non-union is this?
3 What is the treatment of choice?

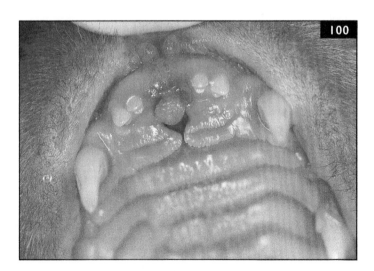

Question 100 This is a 2-year-old cat with a history of chronic sneezing (**100**).
1 What is the midline palatal structure, and what is the cleft?
2 What are possible treatment options?

Answer 99

1 The body of the left mandible is edentulous and appears osteopenic. The alveolar margin has receded and is in close proximity to the mandibular canal, suggesting previous periodontitis. There is a large defect in the area of the missing mandibular first molar tooth. Fracture edges appear smooth with some solid periosteal reaction at the ventral margin.

2 This is a defect non-union fracture in the Weber-Čěch classification of non-union. In this type a critical-size defect is present, which is a defect so large that the body is unable to bridge it, even if the fracture fragments are stabilized.

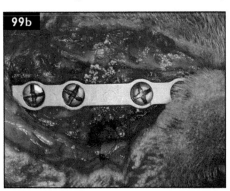

3 Open reduction and internal fixation using a miniplate and screws is indicated, preferably with a titanium locking miniplate (99b). Temporary maxillomandibular fixation may be used to maintain occlusion during the repair. The fracture edges should be débrided. A cancellous bone graft should be applied or, as in this case, a compression-resistant matrix impregnated with rhBMP-2 to stimulate new bone formation and fill in the defect.

Answer 100

1 The round structure on the midline is the incisive papilla; buccal (lateral) are the orifices of the incisive ducts. The incisive ducts communicate with the paired vomeronasal organs and then caudodorsally through the palatine fissures with the nasal cavity. The vomeronasal organs consist of olfactory membrane located at the rostral base of the nasal septum. Lip curling and the 'flehmen response' as a result of sniffing are thought to be a response to open the incisive papilla to allow more molecules to enter and be exposed to the tissue lining the vomeronasal organ. Impulses from the stimulation of this olfactory membrane eventually travel to areas of the hypothalamus associated with sexual and feeding behavior, and possible social interactions. Clients will often ask about the incisive papilla, thinking that this is a tumor in formation. In this case, there are clefts resulting from abnormally wide openings of the incisive ducts. These clefts allow food and other debris to be trapped.

2 Treatment options include increased home hygiene, surgery and an obturator. Increased home hygiene could include the use of instruments to remove the foreign material, or water irrigation either via a curved-tip syringe or Waterpik™. This would require dedication on the part of the client. Surgical options include the use of a sliding flap, pedicle flap, or inverting palatal flap. The risk of this procedure is that the surgery could make the condition worse.

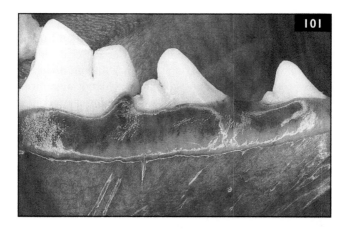

Question 101 The oral cavity is lined by a continuous mucous membrane (**101**).
1 What is the difference between free and attached gingiva?
2 What are the structural differences between attached gingiva, alveolar mucosa, and palatal mucosa?

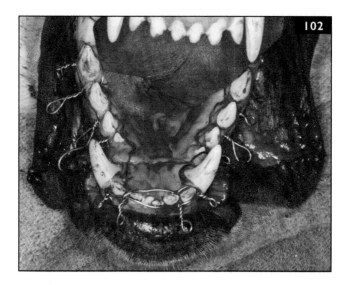

Question 102
1 Name the common types of interdental wiring (**102**).
2 When is interdental wiring indicated?

101, 102: Answers

Answer 101

1 Gingiva covers the alveolar processes of the maxilla and mandible and surrounds the teeth. The gingival mucosa comprises the oral gingival epithelium, sulcular epithelium, and junctional epithelium with the underlying connective tissue (lamina propria) contributing to the attachment apparatus of the tooth (see **110** and **181**). The gingiva coronal to the cementoenamel junction is called the marginal or free gingiva.

2 The attached gingiva is demarcated from the alveolar mucosa by the mucogingival junction and is tightly bound to the underlying periosteum of the alveolar bone. The oral gingival epithelium has a keratinized surface layer. Parakeratinization, characterized by the presence of pyknotic nuclei in the flat, horny scales, is common. The basal cells continuously produce new epithelial cells. The oral gingival epithelium and the lamina propria are dove-tailed with one another through pegs and ridges. The network of collagen fibers in the subepithelial connective tissue, which forms bundles, extends into cementum, periosteum, and the surface of the outer cortical plate of the alveolar process.

The alveolar mucosa is a loose, movable, highly vascularized, non-keratinized epithelium. Compared with the oral gingiva, the connective tissue consists of a submucosa located below the lamina propria. Collagen and elastic fibers are present and the latter give the oral mucosa its mobility. The mucosa of the lips and cheeks and the mucosa of the floor of the mouth are similar in structure to that of the oral mucosa. The epithelium of the mucosa of the floor of the mouth is very thin.

The mucosa of the hard palate consists of keratinized, stratified, squamous epithelium. It is developed in several transverse curved ridges (palatine rugae). It has a thick, tough, connective tissue support, the mucoperiosteum, which is continuous with the periodontal ligaments of the maxillary teeth.

Answer 102

1 Ivy, Stout (as illustrated in **102**), Essig, and Risdon wiring. Ivy loop and Stout multiple-loop techniques are the most commonly used. Both involve a straight run of 22- to 26-gauge wire on the buccal aspect of the teeth, with the other arm of the wire running on the lingual aspect of the teeth. The lingual arm has loops of wire extending buccally between the teeth: a pretwisted loop into which the buccal wire is threaded in the Ivy loop and a single loop placed around the buccal wire in the Stout multiple loop.

2 Rarely is interdental wiring sufficient as the only stabilization for fracture repair. It is much more common now to use an intraoral composite splint, with the interdental wiring used merely as an adjunct to help reinforce the splint. Wiring the teeth together helps maintain occlusion in highly comminuted fractures. It can also help to stabilize the fracture fragments during the building of composite splints.

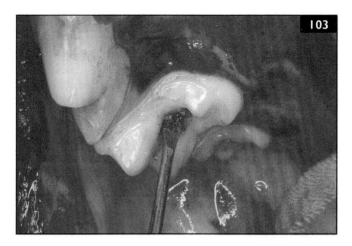

Question 103 This brown lesion on the occlusal surface of this dog's maxillary first molar tooth is leathery and can largely be curetted from the tooth (**103**). Which classic restorative material has historically been used for restoration, and why?

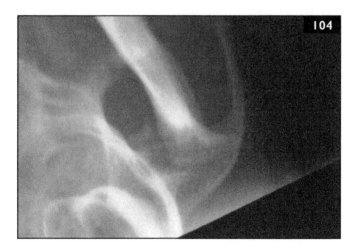

Question 104 This 4-year-old cat was still not eating well 10 days after an apparently well-performed repair of a mandibular symphysis separation (**104**).
1 What is your diagnosis?
2 What imaging modality would be preferred?
3 How common is this type of injury?
4 What are the treatment options?

Answer 103 Treatment of dental caries involves removal of the diseased tooth material, creating an appropriate preparation for the restorative material, and then restoring the lost dental structure. For G.V. Black Class I lesions (occlusal surface of molar teeth or premolar teeth), amalgam still provides excellent properties for restoration. The occlusal table surfaces of these teeth sustain huge compressive forces and no other restorative material matches the strength of amalgam under compressive loads. Typical compressive strength of amalgam (7 days after placement) ranges from 350–500 MPa (50,000–70,000 psi). Also, amalgam is easy to use and is less technique-sensitive than many other materials. It does require removal of slightly more tooth structure to create an undercut for mechanical retention. This retentive undercut may be small, made with a small round or pear-shaped bur. A round or pear-shaped bur undercut avoids a sharp line-angle between the cavity wall and cavity floor, which would introduce a stress point and a space which is difficult to fill. If a bonding agent is not used, the cavity preparation should be lined with a cavity varnish. The amalgam is triturated to mix the mercury with the other metals (i.e. silver, tin, copper, and possibly zinc or palladium). The amalgam is immediately placed into the defect and condensed. Condensation removes voids and bonds the amalgam into a homogenous mass with minimal porosity and residual mercury. Removing excess mercury strengthens the final amalgam by helping to reduce the γ_2-phase (the tin–mercury component which is the weakest). Amalgams with zinc must be protected from moisture contamination by saliva or contaminated instruments. Any water present will react with the zinc, liberating hydrogen gas. Entrapped gas can cause a delayed expansion beginning one week after insertion. This is one reason why zinc-containing amalgams should not be used for retrograde filling following apicoectomy. Once the amalgam is placed, it is carved to the desired shape and the surface and margins are smoothed by burnishing with a ball burnisher. Final polishing should be delayed at least 24 hours.

Answer 104
1 There is an intra-articular fracture of the condylar process of the mandible.
2 Computed tomography with tridimensional reconstruction is the modality of choice.
3 It has been found that this type of injury is relatively common, as mandibular fractures in the cat mainly involve the rostral and the caudal part, contrary to the dog where the body of the mandible is most commonly affected. However, these lesions can easily be overlooked as excellent radiographic technique is required to diagnose them, hence the recommendation to use computed tomography.
4 Because of the limited size of the fracture fragments, internal fixation would prove very difficult, if not impossible. These fractures may heal as a pain-free and functional non-union. Intra-articular or comminuted fractures, however, are likely to result in temporomandibular joint ankylosis; this complication is characterized by a progressive inability to open the mouth (see **117**). Alternatively, a condylectomy, i.e. the surgical removal of the condylar process, can be performed.

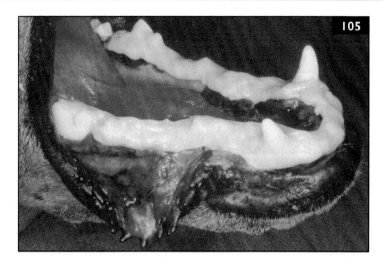

Question 105 What are the indications, advantages, disadvantages, and principles of application of intraoral composite splint fixation of mandibular fractures (105)?

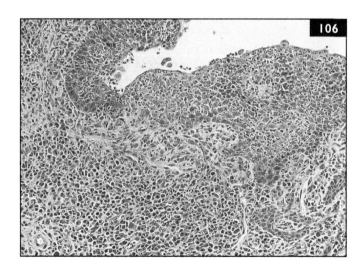

Question 106 Chronic gingivostomatitis in the cat is also known as lymphocytic–plasmacytic gingivostomatitis.
1 What does the term lymphocytic–plasmacytic refer to (106)?
2 Is it of clinical value to biopsy these lesions?

105, 106: Answers

Answer 105 Indications for intraoral composite splint fixation of mandibular fractures include unilateral or bilateral, relatively stable fractures of the mandible, e.g. a fracture between the canine and first premolar teeth. There must be at least two teeth on each side of the fracture which are stable and large enough to provide adequate support (105). One advantage is firm fixation on the tension surface of the fractured bone. Also, the procedure is less invasive than most other options.

The biggest disadvantage of composite splint fixation is the gingivitis which inevitably accompanies the areas covered by the splint. Food, debris, and bacteria accumulate and irritate the tissues. Flushing helps and the gingivitis generally resolves quickly following splint removal.

To apply an intraoral composite splint, the mouth is flushed with a 0.05–0.12% chlorhexidine solution, and the teeth are thoroughly cleaned and polished with pumice polish. They are then acid-etched, rinsed well, and dried. Interdental wiring techniques can be used in conjunction. The composite restorative (e.g. ProTemp Garant, 3M Espe) is then applied incrementally to the etched surfaces. The fracture must be held in reduction and with proper alignment to provide normal occlusion until the composite has set. Then it should be checked for any sharp edges which could irritate the tongue or gingiva. The splint can be built up slightly on the buccal aspect as far caudal as the mandibular fourth premolar tooth. On the mandibular first molar tooth, any build-up must be on the lingual aspect to avoid occlusal interference.

Answer 106

1 Pathologists typically emphasize the types of inflammatory cells that accumulate in oral mucosal lesions. This may create the impression among clinicians that 'lymphocytic–plasmacytic' gingivostomatitis is a specific disease entity in the cat.

Acute lesions are mainly associated with polymorphonuclear neutrophilic infiltrates, whereas increasing numbers and proportions of lymphocytes and plasma cells indicate chronicity. Plasma cells indicate antigenic stimulation. The presence of eosinophils is suggestive of either parasitic or allergic (type-1 hypersensitivity) reactions. Secondary microbial infection is common in oral lesions and results in a mixed inflammatory response. Acute inflammation will have a predominance of neutrophils, whereas chronic inflammation will be characterized by the presence of macrophages, lymphocytes, and plasma cells.

2 Although the histopathologic findings may be consistent with a specific disease process, such as an eosinophilic granuloma, the inflammatory response of oral tissue is often non-specific. A biopsy of feline chronic gingivostomatitis demonstrates a severe and diffuse plasmacytic–lymphocytic infiltrate in deeper tissues and a more ulcerative and suppurative process superficially. With ulcerative lesions in the oral cavity of the cat there is always the possibility of neoplasia, which warrants obtaining a biopsy.

Question 107 This is a late 2-year-old horse (107).
1 What corrective dental procedures are indicated?
2 What is the eruption sequence of the permanent premolar teeth?

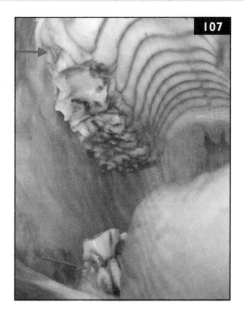

Question 108 This radiograph (108) shows a potential complication of an endodontic procedure.
1 What is the complication evident on this radiograph, and why can this be a problem?
2 What can be done to help prevent this or similar instrument complications?
3 When this complication occurs, what steps can be taken to correct it?

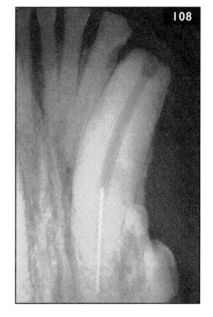

Answer 107

1 Persistent deciduous second premolar teeth are present. These should be extracted as there is a clean demarcation between the deciduous and permanent teeth (red arrows). When a gingival attachment is noted a sulcular incision should be made. Care should be taken to deliver the tooth without separating root tips. The distal portion of the deciduous tooth generally has the most attachment present. A thin molar spreader can be used in the interproximal space distal to the tooth as this will provide elevation. The tooth is grasped with a dental forceps and rolled lingually. Current tetanus vaccine status should be confirmed.

2 A good guideline for eruption of the premolar teeth is: Second premolar teeth: 2 years, 8 months. Third premolar teeth: 2 years, 10 months. Fourth premolar teeth: 3 years, 8 months.

Answer 108

1 The radiograph shows a separated Lentulo® paste filler tip in the root canal. This can be a problem if the presence of the tip prevents adequate obturation of the canal or becomes forced through the apex during obturation. This canal has been previously cleaned since this complication occurred during placement of the root canal cement. If an endodontic file tip becomes separated during the filing stage of the root canal, it may make it impossible to completely clean and shape the canal.

2 Measures to prevent separation of instrument tips during a root canal procedure include: (1) Having a straight-line access to minimize bending of the instrument. (2) Starting with the smallest file that will go to the apical limit of the canal and increasing in size. (3) Using a lubricating agent and lavage during filing. (4) Checking files and spiral filling instruments for signs of weakening (unraveling of the twists or cracks). (5) Keeping a steady hand so the instrument is moved straight in and out of the canal. (6) Using the instrument appropriately (e.g. do not twist Hedström files; use a reduction contra-angle with spiral fillers). (7) Using nickel-titanium files, which are more resistant to separation.

3 If a separated instrument tip does occur, the procedure may still be able to be salvaged. An attempt can be made to remove the instrument tip by using a magnetized file, specialized instrument or ultrasonic endodontic files to loosen and flush the tip out, or try to snag the instrument with another file if in a larger canal. If the tip becomes wedged, it can be impossible to remove it. If the canal is clean and the complication occurred later in the procedure, it may be possible to fill the canal with a heated gutta-percha technique and follow it along radiographically. If there is failure of the procedure or the separated instrument tip prevents satisfactory completion of the root canal procedure, an apicoectomy can be performed to ensure a clean and filled apical portion of the canal.

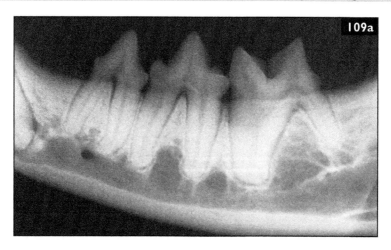

Question 109
1 What is the round radiolucency located ventrally to the mandibular third premolar tooth in this cat (109a)?
2 Where can similar radiolucencies be found in the dog and cat?
3 Which nerves and blood vessels are associated with these structures?

Question 110
1 What are the components of the periodontium?
2 List the periodontal structures marked A–H in 110.
3 What are the ultrastructural characteristics of the junctional epithelium?

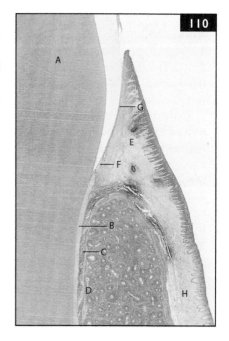

Answer 109
1 A mental foramen.
2 There are usually three mental foramina, both in the dog (**109b**, arrows) and the cat. The middle mental foramen is the main one and is located ventrally to the mesial root of the second premolar tooth in the dog. In the cat, the middle mental foramen is usually located distal to the apex of the canine tooth. A smaller mental foramen is found further caudally, opposite the third premolar tooth. A third mental foramen is situated in the incisive part, at the level of the apex of the second incisor tooth, but this foramen can usually not be seen radiologically.

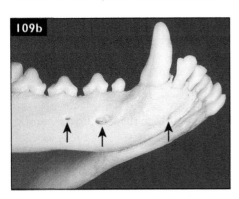

3 The mental nerves are branches of the inferior alveolar nerve which branches from the mandibular nerve. The mental nerves are sensory to the lower lip and the skin of the rostral intermandibular region. The caudal mental artery, middle mental artery, and rostral mental artery and associated veins accompany the mental nerves. The middle mental artery is the largest of the three.

Answer 110
1 Gingiva, periodontal ligament, cementum, and alveolar bone.
2 (A) Dentin. (B) Cementum. (C) Periodontal ligament. (D) Alveolar bone. (E) Gingival connective tissue. (F) Junctional epithelium. (G) Sulcular epithelium. (H) Attached gingiva.
3 Cells of the junctional epithelium (JE) migrate in the direction of their long axis towards the bottom of the sulcus where they are shed. The cells approaching the sulcus contain lysosomes and can phagocytize microorganisms. At the bottom of the sulcus, all JE cells exfoliate and neutrophils can also be seen migrating through the JE. The replacement rate of the JE is about 5 days, which is twice as high as that of the oral gingival epithelium. Subsequently, the desquamation rate is also higher. In contrast to other stratified squamous epithelium of the oral cavity, the JE is only composed of two layers, the active basal layer and an inactive suprabasal layer. The cells all have basically the same structure; they do not undergo a differentiation process like the cells of a keratinized, stratified squamous epithelium. The attachment between the JE and the tooth surface is called the epithelial attachment. This attachment is provided by hemidesmosomes between the tooth surface (covered by acellular afibrillar cementum or by the dental cuticle) and the internal basal lamina developing on the surface of the JE cells in contact with this non-epithelial substrate.

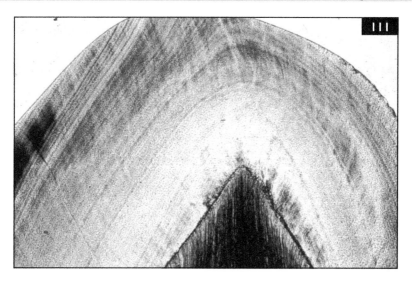

Question 111 Dental enamel is the hardest tissue in the body.
1 How does it differ from other body tissues (**111**)?
2 What are its principal components (also compared with dentin and cementum)?

Question 112 It is important for the veterinary dentist to use correct odontological nomenclature. What are the correct terms to describe the dentition of the dog, horse, and rabbit?

Question 113 A 10-year-old, male castrated Welsh corgi was presented for massive acute blood hemorrhage from the mouth. The clients reported that they woke up to find their dog bleeding. There is no history of trauma, poisoning, or ill-health. Conscious oral examination revealed active hemorrhage seemingly coming from the caudal right mandible, but due to the severe pooling of blood, the exact location of the bleeding could not be identified in the awake patient. Initial laboratory tests (complete blood count, platelet count, serum chemistry panel), including a coagulation profile, were within normal limits.
1 What is your initial assessment of this patient?
2 What is the appropriate plan of action?

Answer 111

1 Enamel is acellular.

2 Enamel is principally composed of closely packed crystals of carbonated calcium hydroxyapatite $[Ca_{10-x}Na_x (PO_4)_{6-y} (CO_3)_2 (OH)_{2-u} F_u]$, aligned as rods or prisms with traces of the protein matrix laid down during enamel formation enveloping each crystal. The composition of enamel, compared with dentin and cementum, is as follows:

	Enamel		Dentin and cementum	
	Weight (%)	Volume (%)	Weight (%)	Volume (%)
Carbonated hydroxyapatite	96	85	70	47
Protein and lipid	1	3	20	33
Water	3	12	10	20

The protein matrix of immature enamel mainly consists of amelogenins, which account for 90% of all enamel proteins. As the enamel matures, amelogenins are broken down by proteinases and the main remaining non-amelogenin proteins include the enamelins. When the teeth of man, primates, and carnivores (where enamel forms the protective covering to the crown) erupt, the enamel is incompletely mineralized. Throughout life there is a constant mineral exchange between the moist oral environment (saliva is normally supersaturated with calcium salts) and enamel, thus allowing the incorporation of fluoride and other ions into the mineral structure. In the presence of fluoride, more fluoroapatite $[Ca_{10}(PO_4)_6F_2]$ is formed, which is less soluble and more acid-resistant than hydroxyapatite. Changes in the oral environment, such as the release of acids during bacterial metabolism within plaque or the application of phosphoric acid 'etchants', can lead to demineralization of enamel. If only the surface layer is affected, remineralization can occur, but since the cells (ameloblasts) which produce enamel have degenerated by the time the tooth erupts into the mouth, enamel cannot repair itself or regenerate when it is otherwise damaged or lost.

Answer 112 *Dog*: a heterodont, diphyodont dentition with anelodont, brachydont teeth. Animals with heterodont dentition have teeth of mixed form and function; being diphyodont, there is a set of primary (deciduous) and secondary (permanent) teeth. Anelodont teeth have a limited period of growth as they develop anatomic roots. In a brachydont dentition the root is longer than the anatomic crown. *Horse*: heterodont, diphyodont and anelodont, like in the dog. However, horses have hypsodont teeth. A hypsodont (radicular hypsodont) tooth has a long anatomic crown and a very short root when fully mature. Much of the crown is held in reserve subgingivally in the alveolar bone. The root is short in comparison with the length of the crown.

Rabbit: heterodont, diphyodont dentition with all teeth being elodont (aradicular hypsodont): elodont teeth grow throughout life and never develop anatomic roots (112). Although diphyodont, the deciduous teeth are not functional and are exfoliated shortly before or after birth.

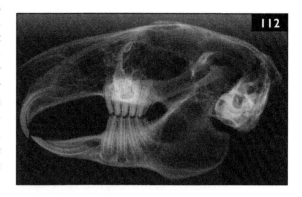

Answer 113

1 The acute and active nature of the bleeding, in light of the normal coagulation profile and platelet count, is suggestive of acute arterial bleeding. An anesthetized oral examination will be necessary to determine the source of the bleeding. The initial packed cell volume (PCV) and total solids (TS) were normal because the time of initial sampling was soon after the hemorrhage started. Serial PCV/TS measurements should be obtained for monitoring purposes. If the source of the hemorrhage is expeditiously identified and controlled, a blood transfusion may not be necessary, but the patient should be blood typed and cross-matched, and a supply of packed RBCs should be readied.

2 Patients, especially smaller-sized patients, with untreated severe periodontal disease may present with acute arterial hemorrhage from the inferior alveolar artery near or at the level of the mandibular first molar tooth, or from the infraorbital artery at the level of the maxillary third to fourth premolar teeth. Tributaries of these larger vessels such as the lateral nasal artery that courses between the maxillary third incisor and canine teeth, and the middle mental artery (113a) are not uncommon sources of significant hemorrhage. The severity of periodontitis-related bone loss leads to exposure and erosion of the artery resulting in profound active hemorrhage, as seen in this case (113b), which leads to immediate action and treatment. Often the presentation is more misleading, where the bleeding is intermittent, resulting in a pattern of active bleeding–clotting–swallowing of blood, such that the patient presents without strikingly notable bleeding, and is subsequently discharged without treatment; only to return on an emergency basis when there is active hemorrhage. Once the source of bleeding is identified, the involved tooth or teeth are extracted, which often provides enough exposure to visualize the bleeding vessel, which can then be ligated. Additional exposure may be necessary, for example a buccal corticotomy may be necessary along the mandible to ligate the inferior alveolar artery, especially if the vessel has been completely transected.

Other sources of acute oral hemorrhage, arising from the same vessels, may develop secondary to oral neoplasia. Hemorrhage of this severity is more typically associated with inoperable oral tumors, and control of the hemorrhage is only attainable by gross debulking of the tumor with flap closure, palliative radiation therapy, or in some cases, interventional therapies such as vascular embolization. Chinese herbs such as Yunnan Baiyao, when used alone or in combination with the mineral phosphorous 30C, may aid in hemorrhage control.

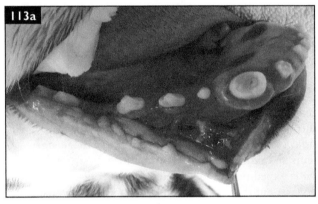

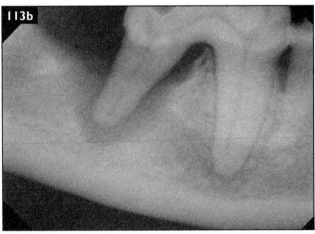

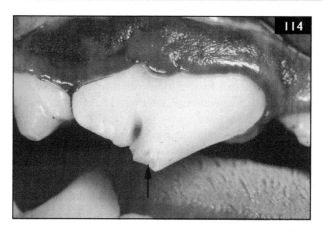

Question 114
1 Why is exposed dentin sensitive, as in this uncomplicated crown fracture (114, arrow)?
2 What generally prevents bacterial access to the pulp when a vital tooth's patent dentinal tubules are exposed?
3 How are these lesions typically addressed?

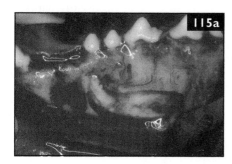 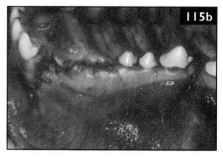

Question 115 Which type of flap is being used for the surgical extraction of this impacted maxillary canine tooth in this dog (in dorsal recumbency) (115a, b)?

Answer 114

1 The 'dentin–pulp complex' is a living tissue. There are presently three theories to explain the sensitivity of dentin. The direct innervation theory is based on the presence of nerve endings alongside many of the odontoblastic processes within dentinal tubules, which can be stimulated directly. These nerve fibers, however, do not extend to the dentinoenamel junction. The hydrodynamic theory, which currently predominates, is based on the belief that fluid movement in the dentinal tubules stimulates the nerve endings. The transduction theory, for which there is less support, is based on the assumption that the odontoblasts act as receptors.

2 Healthy pulp is enclosed within a solid casing, the tooth. Pulpal blood vessels are thin-walled so that pressure within the pulp is at or near to arterial blood pressure. This pressure is sufficient to force tissue fluid to flow out through patent dentinal tubules which are exposed on the tooth surface. Under natural circumstances, air and fluid pressure within the oral cavity rarely match this pressure, so bacteria have difficulty entering the pulp. Provided that the odontoblasts have not been irreparably damaged, the exposed dentinal tubules become sclerotic and are sealed by the progressive formation of intratubular dentin.

3 Recently exposed dentinal tubules can be sealed with bonding agents or dentin desensitizers.

Answer 115 Pedicle flaps can be created to accommodate almost any tooth or group of teeth by making releasing incisions at either end of an envelope flap, then extending the gingival and periosteal elevation, usually creating a mucogingival flap (115c). The periosteum on the under-surface of full-thickness mucogingival flaps is inelastic. By incising through the periosteum without damaging the

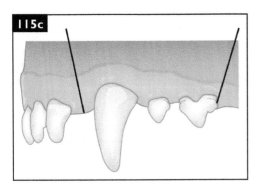

115c

under-surface of the mucosa, it is possible to produce a much more mobile tissue flap which can be advanced over tissue defects such as oronasal fistulas. The most important aspect of flap closure is first, to avoid any tension on the closure, and second, to avoid having unsupported suture lines. Whenever possible the suture line should be over healthy bone or soft tissue, not over a void.

Question 116 This dog has had a traumatic injury to its maxillary canine tooth (**116**).

1 What are the differences between an avulsed tooth, a luxated tooth, and a subluxated tooth?
2 What would be an appropriate treatment plan to salvage this tooth?
3 When is endodontic therapy appropriate for these teeth?

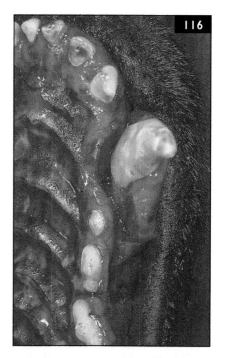

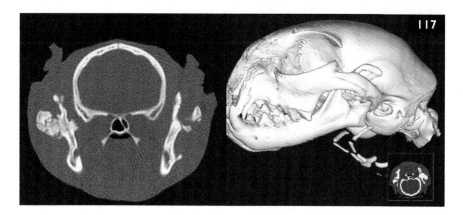

Question 117 This cat was hit by a car and developed a progressive inability to open its mouth (**117**).

1 What is your diagnosis?
2 What is the treatment, aftercare, and prognosis?

Answer 116

1 An avulsed (or exarticulated) tooth is one that has become completely separated from the alveolus. These teeth must be reimplanted soon after the injury, ideally within 30 minutes, as damage to the periodontal ligament attachment occurs from desiccation. The prognosis is guarded and some tooth resorption is likely.

A luxated tooth is one that has lateral, intrusive or extrusive displacement. The tooth shown in (116) has significant lateral displacement disrupting the buccal alveolar wall. There will be significant mobility and a luxated tooth will not remain stable when replaced in its alveolus. A luxated tooth has a better prognosis than a completely avulsed tooth.

A subluxated tooth is one that has become mobile from a traumatic injury but has not become displaced. It may not need to be stabilized to allow repair of the periodontal ligament.

2 A treatment plan for a laterally luxated tooth is to obtain an intraoral radiograph to evaluate the hard tissues, and gently débride the palatal alveolar area and root surface. The periodontal ligament fibers should be left intact if they appear healthy. The tooth is replaced into the alveolus and stabilized. Several options are available to stabilize this tooth depending upon the degree of mobility and presence of anchor teeth. A figure-of-eight wire around the two maxillary canine teeth stabilized with acrylic or composite resin material is a simple method to stabilize a canine tooth that has instability laterally and a healthy counterpart. An acrylic or composite resin splint can be placed between several adjacent teeth in the same arch to obtain good stability also. The splint may be left in place for 4–6 weeks. Endodontic treatment is performed as described below and the tooth is followed radiographically to determine continued treatment success. Signs of failure include root resorption and ankylosis.

3 Endodontic treatment is generally required in avulsed and luxated teeth due to the disruption of the blood supply to the tooth and subsequent pulp death. Various times have been recommended for endodontic treatment. The current recommendation is that root canal therapy should be done 10–20 days after initial treatment. Avulsed teeth that are treated endodontically at the time of reimplantation may have a worse prognosis.

Answer 117

1 This is a case of pseudo-ankylosis of the temporomandibular joint, likely due to osteophyte formation as a post-traumatic complication, resulting in a bony bridge between the coronoid process of the mandible and the zygomatic arch. This differs from true ankylosis, where the bony fusion is located within the temporomandibular joint.

2 Treatment consists of excision of all osteophytes or segmental caudal mandibulectomy. A condylectomy is indicated if the actual joint is involved. Aftercare should ensure plenty of chewing activity, by feeding large-size kibble and providing chew-toys to prevent re-ankylosis. The prognosis is guarded to poor, as the cut bony surfaces are inclined to re-ankylose.

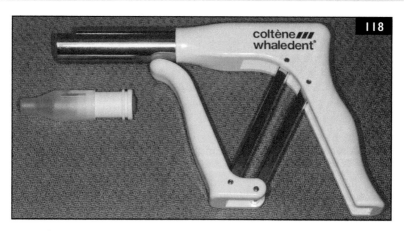

Question 118

1 This dispenser and capsule (**118**) are used for what gutta-percha technique?
2 How is this product used?
3 What are the advantages of this gutta-percha technique over other traditional techniques?

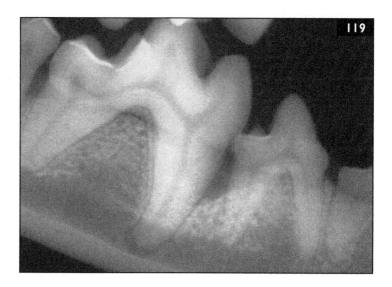

Question 119

1 Describe the radiologic findings on this radiograph (**119**).
2 How would you determine whether the described lesions are associated with disease?

Answer 118

1 This is a proprietary dispenser designed for the application of cold flowable self-curing gutta-percha and sealer (GuttaFlow2®, Coltène Whaledent, Inc.) which is used as a root canal obturation material. GuttaFlow® incorporates a <30 µm gutta-percha particle size with a polydimethylsiloxane sealer into an easy-to-use flowable product. The product is provided in capsules that are mixed in a standard triturator for 30 seconds. Regular- (25–30 minutes) and fast-set (8–10 minutes) versions of the product are available.

2 GuttaFlow® is syringed directly into the canal using tips, or indirectly with a paste filler or with a GuttaFlow®-coated gutta-percha cone or paper point. Because the canal tips included with the product are short, 25 mm in length, they are best used for shorter, wider canals; therefore when a longer-length tip is desirable, for example with a canine tooth in a dog, intravenous catheter sleeves may facilitate apical obturation. The product may be used as a sole obturation material, but is typically used as a backfill material in combination with single-cone techniques that use a master gutta-percha cone or apical gutta-percha plug (SimpliFill® Apical Plugs, SybronEndo Corporation).

3 GuttaFlow® does not require heat, is cold curing, has good dimensional stability, and may actually expand slightly. Shrinkage is not a concern with GuttaFlow® as it is with thermoplastic gutta-percha products when they cool, which is particularly useful when obturating wide canals in young animals. Because GuttaFlow® is a combination of gutta-percha and sealer it adheres directly to dentin and gutta-percha itself, which helps to reduce procedural time. By its very nature as a flowable product, it has excellent flow characteristics for negotiating tight/curved canals and filling accessory canals. A flowable product such as GuttaFlow® also does not require compaction.

Answer 119

1 Vertical bone loss resulting in a deep infrabony pocket is evident on the mesial aspect of the mesial root of the right mandibular first molar tooth, also involving the distal root of the fourth premolar tooth. In addition, there is a distinct periapical radiolucent area associated with the former root. This lesion may be normal anatomy or represent pathology. Where it represents normal anatomy, it is a radiographic artifact due to the root apex dipping into the mandibular canal or lying in close proximity to the canal. Where it represents pathology, it is an extension of a chronic pulpitis or an inflammatory reaction due to pulpal necrosis.

2 The infrabony pocket can be confirmed by periodontal probing and is associated with the presence of periodontitis. The fact that the periapical radiolucency appears to be an extension of the root shape, rather than a round ballooning lesion, is suggestive for normal anatomy. Comparison should always be made with other teeth of the same type in the same animal. A contralateral radiograph is indicated, particularly if the tooth seems healthy, e.g. no sign of crown fracture or pulpal involvement, on clinical examination.

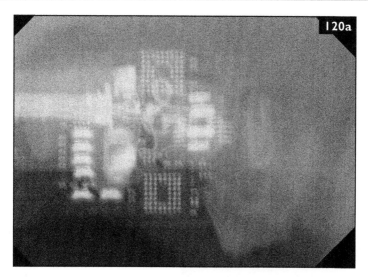

Question 120
1 What is the cause of the artifact seen on this digital dental radiograph (120a)?
2 What other errors can occur with digital dental radiographic techniques that can make images difficult to evaluate?

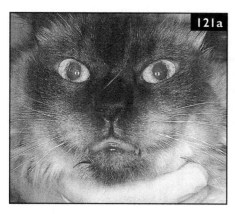 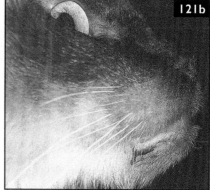

Question 121
1 What endocrinopathy should be considered in a cat with insulin-resistant diabetes mellitus, hepatomegaly, and a large head with a protruding mandible (121a, b)?
2 What would be the most likely cause, and how would the diagnosis be confirmed?

Answer 120

1 The digital sensor was positioned backwards in the mouth and the incorrect side of the sensor was exposed to the incoming X-ray beam. The exposure surface of rigid charge-coupled device (CCD) digital sensors is flat, whereas the opposite surface of the sensor is not flat, as it includes the wire insertion point into the sensor, making the occurrence of this artifact infrequent.

2 Although rigid CCD digital sensors cannot be bent, phosphor plates can, and similar to traditional dental film, where the emulsion of the film can be damaged by rough handling – bent, creased with a sharp fingernail when removing the packet from the film, scratched with an X-ray clip, or damaged from the cusp of a tooth – phosphor plates can also be scratched, creased, bent or folded, and these artifacts will reveal themselves when the plates are scanned, compromising the image quality (120b). Under- and overexposed digital images can typically be corrected using the image enhancement tools

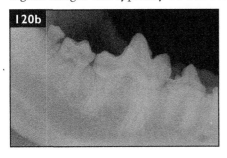

included with digital radiography software without having to retake the image. Since CCD digital sensors and phosphor plate films cannot be sterilized, proper infection control protocols should be followed in accordance with manufacturer instructions for covering and cleaning CCD sensors between patients.

Answer 121

1 Chronic hypersecretion of growth hormone (GH) results in acromegaly. Growth hormone excesses induce peripheral insulin resistance. Other clinical features that may be present include cardiomegaly, congestive heart failure, nephromegaly, nephropathy (proteinuria, azotemia), renal failure, weight gain/loss, body enlargement, arthropathy, large tongue, and central nervous system signs.

2 A GH-secreting tumor of the pituitary gland is the most common cause of acromegaly in cats. Hyperadrenocorticism and hyperthyroidism are other endocrinopathies that may be associated with insulin-resistant diabetes and they should be excluded in the diagnostic evaluation of an insulin-resistant diabetic cat. Demonstrating significantly elevated circulating GH concentrations is diagnostic for acromegaly; however, there is limited availability of veterinary laboratories performing feline GH assays. Indirect evaluation of GH concentration by measuring somatomedin C (insulin-like growth factor-1) may be beneficial. A presumptive diagnosis of acromegaly is made when the thyroid and adrenal glands are normal and the cat has characteristic clinical signs and laboratory data, and a pituitary mass is identified. Computed tomography (CT) or magnetic resonance imaging (MRI) may be used to demonstrate a pituitary mass.

Question 122
1 What is the clinical diagnosis in this 5-year-old rabbit (**122a**) presented for weight loss?
2 Is this a common condition and what is the underlying pathophysiology?
3 What should the diagnostic work-up entail?

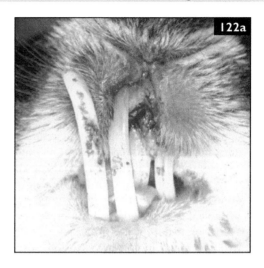

Question 123 Halitosis in pets is a very common complaint among pet owners.
1 What conditions may cause halitosis? What is their respective importance?
2 How is halitosis produced?
3 How can it be assessed?
4 How can it be treated?

Question 124
1 Discuss the use of a piezoelectric scaler in veterinary dentistry (**124a**).
2 Besides professional scaling, what are other dental applications where piezoelectric technology can be applied?
3 Describe the use of piezoelectric technology in clinical oromaxillofacial surgery; what are the benefits of piezosurgery versus conventional mechanical or electrical instruments for this purpose?

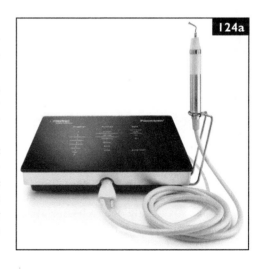

Answer 122

1 Incisor malocclusion with associated soft-tissue trauma to the lips is evident.

2 Incisor malocclusion is relatively common in rabbits. If this condition occurs as an isolated entity at an early age, it is probably due to maxillary brachygnathia, which is of genetic origin. Because of the abnormal incisor occlusion, insufficient attrition takes place resulting in excessive overgrowth of the incisor teeth. The maxillary incisor teeth, with their inherently greater curvature, typically curl into the oral cavity, while the mandibular incisor teeth grow in a dorsofacial direction. If left untreated, trauma to the lip, palate and other maxillofacial structures may occur.

A total lack of dietary material for gnawing may also result in incisor overgrowth. Incisor overgrowth may occur subsequent to the loss or fracture of an opposing incisor tooth. Fracture of an incisor tooth may result in pulpal necrosis, periapical disease and cessation of growth and eruption.

Incisor malocclusion may also be secondary to, or occurring concomitantly with, premolar-molar malocclusion. Conversely, incisor malocclusion may lead to premolar-molar malocclusion. In fact, incisor malocclusion without premolar-molar abnormalities may be relatively rare.

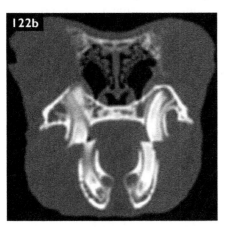

3 Because of the likelihood of the incisor malocclusion being part of a more generalized malocclusion, rabbits with incisor malocclusion should always receive a comprehensive oral examination under general examination and appropriate diagnostic imaging. Computed tomography (122b) is especially useful for showing the premolar and molar occlusion and periapical changes, without the problem of superposition of dental quadrants encountered with conventional radiography.

Answer 123

1 Halitosis may have extraoral and oral causes. Extraoral causes are related to diet (e.g. garlic in humans), metabolic diseases (diabetes, uremia), and infections (respiratory infections, e.g. pneumonia). Halitosis originating from the oral cavity is mostly due to bacterial activity in the mouth. It can be enhanced by oral tissue destruction during disease, by oral stagnation of food, and by stagnation of saliva in a specific area (e.g. lip fold) as well as by reduction of salivary flow. Halitosis is associated with oral causes in 85% of people affected. Periodontal disease is a very common cause of halitosis. Gastric conditions are

not a common cause of halitosis as gas cannot come out from the stomach, except during the process of belching.

2 Halitosis of extraoral origin is due to the presence of malodorous substances in the bloodstream which pass through the alveolar membrane of the lungs into the respired air. These substances may have a metabolic origin or a digestive origin (food). Halitosis originating from the mouth is due to the production of malodorous volatile gas by the putrefactive action of bacteria on exogenous and endogenous protein substrates such as exfoliated epithelium, salivary components, food debris, and blood. Anaerobes (especially Gram-negatives) associated with periodontal disease produce volatile sulfur compounds (VSCs), such as particularly hydrogen sulfide and mercaptan, which are responsible for bad breath.

3 Halitosis is commonly assessed by organoleptic methods. With subjective methods, it is generally accepted that three levels (weak, moderate, strong) can be recognized. However, this is not accurate, especially if assessment of the same dog over a period of time or comparison between dogs is necessary. The use of a panel of 'blind' examiners has been shown effective in halitosis research. Selection, calibration, and training of the examiners is necessary for optimal results. An objective method based on the measurement of VSCs with an electrochemical sensor (Halimeter® (**123a**)) has been shown accurate and reliable. Orastrip® (**123b**) measures VSCs and high levels are believed to be associated with active bacterial activity and periodontitis.

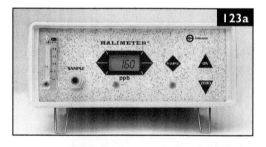

4 Recent studies in dogs using organoleptic methods for measuring halitosis have demonstrated a significant decrease in halitosis in dogs that received a daily oral gel (Tooth to Tail®) containing a synergistic combination of essential oils and polyphenolic antioxidants. Essential oils such as menthol and thymol have a documented antibacterial effect; while the addition of pure plant-derived antioxidants (phloretin and ferulic acid) balances oxidative stress by neutralizing free radicals and reactive oxygen species (ROS) associated with bacterial-induced inflammation.

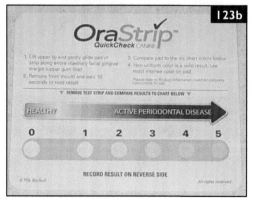

Answer 124

1 Piezoelectric scalers are popular in Asia and Europe, are steadily gaining ground in the States, and are the most common type of stock power scaler included on mobile dental delivery units. The ultrasonic activity is created by high-frequency currents that are applied to ceramic discs or quartz plates within the handpiece – pressure electrification. The tip motion of piezoelectric scalers is linear ranging from 25–50 thousand cycles per second. Less heat is generated from piezoelectric scalers; therefore, less water lavage is needed during scaling. Piezoelectric scalers are typically quieter than magnetostrictive scalers, and have ergonomic wide-diameter handpieces. Many units also have the option of fiberoptic or LED (light-emitting diode) lighting.

2 Another benefit of the majority of traditional piezoelectric scalers is that they are true multifunction units that with a simple change of the scaler tip and the power setting can be transformed from a scaler to an instrument useful for endodontic surgery – apicoectomy, apicoectomy retrograde preparations, and even as a device for retrieving root tips/separated root canal files.

3 Specialized piezosurgery units are available that allow for cutting of bone and performing surgical tooth extractions. These units are more than simply dental piezoelectric units with an increased power supply: in addition to having more power, they allow for selective cutting of bone relative to soft tissues (vessels, nerves and mucosa), provide a clear surgical field from irrigation and hemostasis/anti-bacterial action associated with cavitation effect, and generate little to no heat, reducing bone necrosis. Piezosurgery is very technique-sensitive, and is influenced by the tip design, pressure applied to the tip, speed

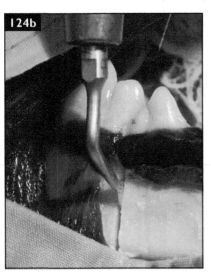

of forward-to-back movement, and also by the density of the bone. For example, bone of high density requires a high-frequency setting and low-density bone requires a lower-frequency setting for maximum cutting efficiency. In veterinary oral surgery, piezosurgery is an excellent instrument to use when performing an odontogenic cyst enucleation, to prevent tearing of the delicate cyst epithelium, and with oral cancer surgery, in particular with mandibulectomies, where use of piezosurgery will minimize the necessary soft-tissue elevation prior to the ostectomy, and will provide protection of the neurovascular bundle (124b).

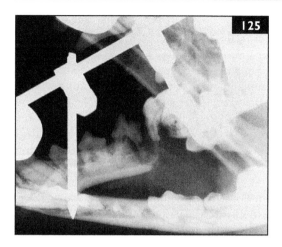

Question 125 This is a 4-month follow-up radiograph of a mandibular fracture stabilized with an external fixator. It indicates that a non-union is present, even though the repair is still very stable (125).
1 What is/are the likely cause(s) of this complication?
2 What are the recommended guidelines for preventing this problem?
3 What would the therapeutic approach be at this stage?

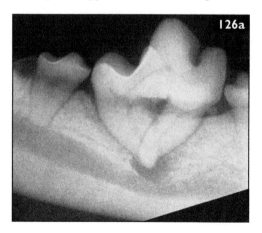

Question 126 This radiograph (126a) illustrates the need for pre-extraction radiographs.
1 Give three examples of changes associated with a tooth where a pre-extraction radiograph is valuable.
2 What other valuable information can be gained from a pre-extraction radiograph of very mobile teeth?

133

Answer 125

1 The distal root of the mandibular fourth premolar tooth and the mesial root of the first molar tooth are involved in the fracture line. These roots are poorly supported by bone, and a severe periodontal–endodontic lesion is present at the distal root of the mandibular fourth premolar tooth. A large bone defect is present, which has also contributed to this non-viable, defect non-union.

2 It is common for an alveolus to be involved in the fracture line. If the tooth involved is luxated, it should be removed. If there is still enough healthy periodontal attachment, evidenced by the fact that the tooth is non-mobile, retention of the tooth is usually indicated as it will contribute to the stability of the fracture fixation. The presence of a tooth in the fracture line increases the incidence of infectious complications; however, the immediate removal of the tooth cannot reverse these effects. If a tooth involved in the fracture line is retained, it should be carefully monitored subsequently for any evidence of periodontal or endodontal pathology; appropriate treatment should be instituted as soon as either is recognized.

3 The two affected teeth should be extracted and the area débrided. Antibiotic therapy, which ideally should be based on bacteriologic examination of a sample taken intraoperatively, is indicated. Once the infection is resolved and inflammation subsided, a mandibular reconstruction using a titanium miniplate and screws, and a bone graft or bone-regenerative approach are indicated.

Answer 126

1 This tooth has an abnormal root structure which will make extraction difficult. The tooth with a normal-appearing crown may have evidence of pathologic root resorption. In cases of persistent deciduous teeth (**126b**), it is important to know whether and to what extent physiologic root resorption has taken place. A fractured crown of a mandibular tooth may show evidence of periapical pathology in close proximity with the ventral margin bone which may result in an iatrogenic fracture when attempting to extract this tooth. Other conditions that

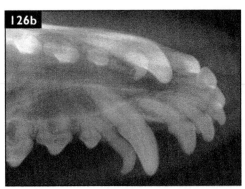

would influence the extraction technique include: supernumerary roots, fused roots, root dilaceration, and root fracture.

2 Tooth mobility leading to extraction of the tooth may be secondary to neoplastic processes or metabolic bone diseases such as hyperparathyroidism. Extensive osteolysis of bone and fractures of the mandible or maxilla may also result in mobility of teeth.

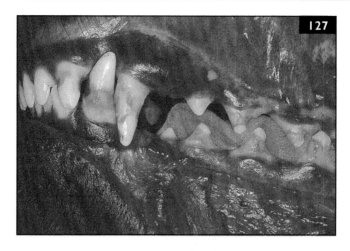

Question 127 What is known about the etiology of the disorder seen here (127)?

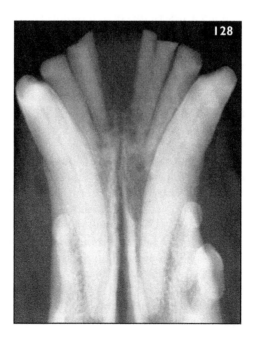

Question 128 What are the radiologic findings associated with this 15-mm diameter, exophytic tumor on the gingival margin of the mandibular first incisor teeth in a dog (128)? In general, how does one systematically evaluate radiographs of suspected oral tumors?

Answer 127 The etiology of enamel hypoplasia is associated with periods of high fever, infections, nutritional deficiencies, disturbances of the metabolism, and systemic disorders. Epitheliotropic viral infection (particularly when caused by morbilliviruses, such as distemper), is the most common cause, and was also the cause in the case depicted. In most cases a differentiation between a generalized disturbance and a local one can be made.

A metabolic disturbance over a longer period during the enamel development will cause generalized enamel defects. Symmetric belt-like defects and discolorations are found on the dentition where the enamel was formed during the systemic disturbance. In cases of generalized enamel defects, all teeth are usually affected. Radiographs should be obtained as root hypoplasia and other malformations can be present.

A metabolic disturbance of short duration during the development of enamel can be recognized by defects limited to a circumscribed area of the affected teeth. Local enamel defects typically occur symmetrically and on homologous teeth. Only those ameloblasts which, at the time of the disturbance, had just started enamel formation are affected. Trauma is a common cause of localized enamel defects.

Answer 128 The radiologic descriptors of oral tumors systematically focus on the appearance of the lesion, surrounding bone, and teeth. In evaluating the lesion, one should note the size, border, density, and number of the lesion(s). In this particular example, there is a single, 15-mm diameter, peripheral, soft-tissue density with ill-defined margins on the bony interface. There is no evidence of mineralization in the tumor. The surrounding bone can show evidence of expansion, perforation, erosion, and remodeling. Ill-defined margins and destruction of the bone cortex are suggestive of a malignancy, while expansion of the cortex is more indicative of a benign lesion (see **14**). With a benign lesion, a layer of smooth reactive bone may be found on the outside. Bone resorption can be focal (or geographical), moth-eaten, or permeative. In this example, there is evidence of a predominantly moth-eaten pattern of bone resorption between the roots of the first incisor teeth and deeper down the left mandible. The rostral mental foramen on that side is markedly enlarged. Teeth involved in an oral tumor can either be in their original position, displaced, or partially resorbed. Displaced teeth, as in this example, are more commonly found in relatively benign tumors, while aggressive, malignant tumors tend to leave the teeth 'floating' in their original position.

This radiograph (**128**) was obtained of a canine acanthomatous ameloblastoma, previously known as an 'acanthomatous epulis'. The radiologic findings associated with odontogenic and non-odontogenic tumors are generally non-specific. However, radiographs form an important part of the clinical staging in determining the extent of the tumor and in establishing whether bone involvement is present. Apparently normal radiographs do not rule out bone infiltration, as about 40% of the bone must be resorbed before this becomes visible using conventional radiography.

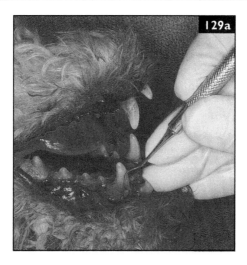

Question 129 Define scaling, root planing, and gingival curettage, and explain how these three procedures may form part of routine periodontal treatment (**129a**).

Question 130
1 What is CAD/CAM restorative dentistry?
2 What are the advantages and disadvantages to CAD/CAM techniques versus traditional techniques?

Question 131 The curette on the right has been sharpened many times incorrectly compared with the curette on the left (**131**).
1 What incorrect sharpening technique has created the pointed tip of the curette on the right?
2 What are three basic sharpening techniques for use on curettes and scalers?
3 What is the proper angle between the face of a curette and the surface of a flat stone?

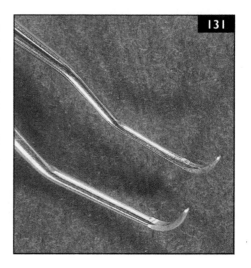

Answer 129 *Scaling* (**129b**, A) is the removal of accretions (plaque and calculus) from the teeth. Scaling implies a procedure to clean the accessible part of the tooth, in order to remove acquired material which is likely to promote the development of disease. It does not signify preparation of the surface involved. When there is severe gingival inflammation, 'gross' scaling is performed to remove the majority of local irritants, with the intent to proceed to more thorough and exacting techniques. The rationale for staging treatment in this manner is that some tissue healing can occur before other more delicate procedures are instituted – usually at least a few days later. The end point in scaling is visual cleanliness. *Root planing* (**129b**, B) is removal of accretions and smoothing the root surface. Root planing may be directed at cementum irregularities or notches left in the tooth surface by previous therapeutic procedures. The end point of root planing is tactile smoothness of the root. An instrument, such as an explorer, is used to feel the root surface. Overlapping short smooth strokes with a sharp periodontal curette are used to create this surface. *Gingival curettage* (**129b**, C) indicates removal of granulation tissue and diseased epithelium from the sulcus or pocket lining by scraping the soft tissue with a curette. A universal curette held in the reverse position from that used for normal scaling can be used for this procedure; a finger held against the gingiva can stabilize the gingiva during the curettage. The operator must exercise discretion in how much pressure to apply in scraping the soft tissue: enough to remove the friable diseased tissue but not so much that the gingiva is badly torn. Gingival curettage is generally performed in a closed fashion, i.e. without creating a gingival flap. The rationale behind this procedure is that the defect created is expected to heal by epithelial regeneration, resulting in long but healthier junctional epithelium and some connective tissue reattachment.

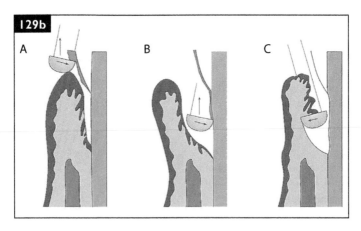

Answer 130

1 CAD/CAM (computer-aided design/computer-aided manufacturing) was introduced to dentistry in the mid-1980s, and uses scanned images of the crown preparation margins to mill the restoration (e.g. full-coverage crown, veneers, inlay or onlay) out of a solid ceramic or composite resin block. Additional stains and glazes are then applied to the milled prosthesis to improve esthetics. Scanning of the margins and surrounding teeth is typically performed using a handheld device (**130a**), and avoids the use of traditional impression materials, but is much more technique sensitive with respect to pre-requisites of a dry field devoid of sulcular moisture/blood, with good separation of the soft and hard tissues from the preparation margins, since there is no impression material to flow into these areas. Use of a diode laser or electrosurgery unit for 'troughing' is preferable to gingival cords to achieve the necessary retraction, visibility, and hemostasis prior to obtaining a CAD/CAM scan. To avoid lens fogging and provide accurate intraoral scans the lens of the handheld scanner is heated with a temperature-adjustable heater plate in the scanner cradle. The digital scans are either transmitted to an authorized outside laboratory through an online portal, or to a chairside milling unit (**130b**) for in-house fabrication of the prosthesis. The computer uses reverse engineering to create a replacement 'part' for the areas of missing tooth (**130c**).

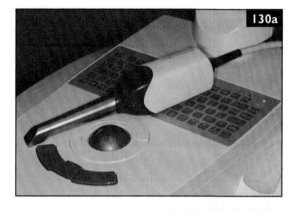

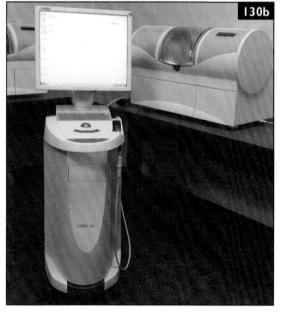

2 CAD/CAM technology offers superior accuracy in comparison to traditional impression techniques and eliminates the impression-taking step, provides a completed prosthesis in a single visit, and removes the need for a provisional restoration. CAD/CAM restorations rival the quality and esthetics of traditional prosthetics, but do not eliminate the artistic license of an experienced dental laboratory technician; without the application of appropriate stains and glazes, the CAD/CAM milled restoration would be unnaturally monochromatic in color. Despite its many identifiable advantages in human dentistry, the high capital investment associated with implementing CAD/CAM technology is likely cost prohibitive for most veterinary dental practices.

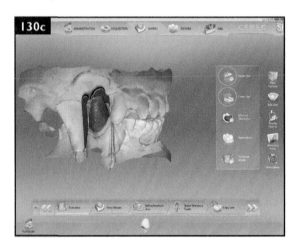

Answer 131

1 A point is created on a curette when too much pressure is placed on the toe of the instrument during sharpening, or when both sides of the instrument are sharpened in this fashion. The entire working tip of the curette should be placed evenly against the stone.

2 (1) The moving flat stone technique: here, the instrument is held securely in the hand off a counter edge or against a sharpening guide. The stone is placed against the working tip in the appropriate angle and then moved steadily in short strokes back and forth against the instrument. (2) The stationary flat stone technique: here, the stone is placed on a solid surface or in a stone holder and the instrument is placed on the stone at the appropriate angle and moved steadily back and forth across the surface. (3) The conical stone method: here, a narrow conical stone is moved in a sweeping stroke across the face of the working tip towards the toe of the curette.

Any of the three techniques can be used successfully if done properly and frequently to maintain sharp instruments.

3 The proper angle formed by the face of the curette when placed on a flat stone and the stone surface is 100–110°.

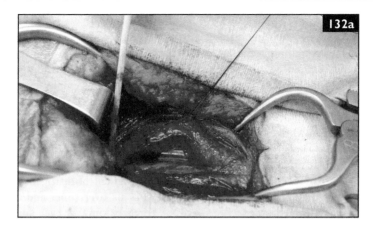

Question 132 In a retrospective study of 20 cats, 70% of tracheal tears in cats were identified as being associated with anesthetized dental procedures (**132a**). Tears to the dorsal membrane are the most common.
1 What are the symptoms of this condition and how is it diagnosed?
2 What is the treatment for tracheal tears?
3 How can this complication be avoided?

Question 133
1 Define host modulation therapy (HMT) for the treatment of refractory periodontal disease.
2 What class of antibiotics has been used for HMT?

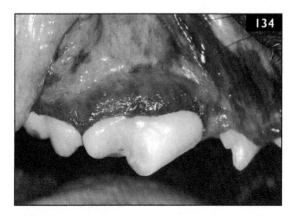

Question 134 Which type of bonding agent would be appropriate for this restoration (**134**)?

Answer 132
1 Tracheal tear symptoms include subcutaneous emphysema, dyspnea, respiratory stridor, coughing, gagging, anorexia, lethargy, vomiting and fever. The condition is diagnosed by recognition of the symptoms and radiography (i.e. documentation of pneumomediastinum and subcutaneous emphysema), and less commonly by tracheoscopy or computed tomography.
2 In cases of iatrogenic rupture of the trachea, supportive care (oxygen therapy and cage rest until the emphysema resolves) is usually all that is necessary, and healing of the rupture occurs spontaneously. Resolution of the emphysema is typically a slow process, and may take as long as 1–6 weeks because reabsorption of the air depends on the small diffusion gradient of nitrogen. With tears closer to the carina, or if the emphysema worsens over time, and/or a pneumothorax develops, thoracocentesis (**132b**), tracheostomy, or even surgery (ventral cervical midline approach with a partial midline sternotomy) to correct the defect may be necessary.

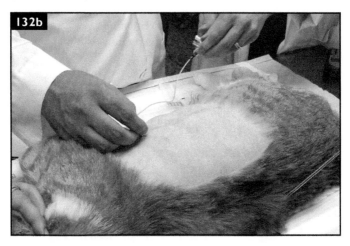

3 The benefits of ensuring a protected airway with a cuffed endotracheal tube in preventing the aspiration of fluids during dental procedures certainly outweigh the risks of tracheal tears; however, several steps should be taken to minimize the risk of tracheal tears, and these include: (1) utilize as large a diameter tube as can be atraumatically accommodated between the arytenoid cartilages; (2) improve the seal of the cuff and facilitate intubation by applying a coating of sterile lubricant onto the cuff; (3) ensure an adequate but safe volume of cuff insufflation by inflating the cuff with no more than 6 mL of air, or with more air than the seal obtained by verifying the absence of a leak (i.e. when the sound of hissing stops) at 20 mmHg inspiratory airway pressure; (4) avoid rotating

the endotracheal tube within the trachea when changing the patient's recumbency–disconnect and reconnect the anesthesia circuit from the tube when rotating the patient; (5) always deflate the cuff before extubating; (6) use of a swivel-type elbow connector for the anesthesia circuit (132c).

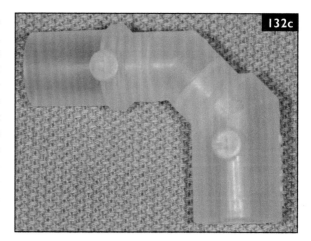

132c

Answer 133

1 Refractory periodontitis is defined as the development of additional sites of attachment loss despite concurrent and repeated attempts to control the periodontitis by traditional methods of treatment. Host modulation therapy or HMT is an emerging concept in the treatment of periodontitis that focuses on the reduction, stabilization, or regeneration of the tissue by modulating the host response and restoring the balance between pro-inflammatory mediators and anti-inflammatory mediators, and is useful as an adjunctive therapy to traditional scaling and root planing (SRP). NSAIDs, bisphosphonates, sub-antimicrobial dose doxycycline (SDD), nitric oxide synthase inhibitors, omega-3 fatty acids, and growth factors are some of the many therapeutic agents that have been investigated with HMT properties. Patients with refractory periodontitis are ideal candidates for HMT.

2 Matrix metalloproteinases or MMPs and are a family of approximately 25 zinc-dependent proteolytic enzymes that are essential to normal tissue homeostasis, and are mediators responsible for extracellular matrix degradation, including collagen type I destruction associated with active periodontitis. MMPs such as MMP-8 are prevalent in diseased saliva and periodontal tissue, and may be useful as biomarkers for periodontal disease. The inhibition of MMP-8 and -13 activity with non-antimicrobial/sub-antimicrobial dose tetracycline and tetracycline analogs has shown promising clinical results (i.e. improvement in clinical attachment level and probing depth) when used in combination with SRP or open flap surgery. Doxycycline hyclate is the only member of the tetracycline family that has been FDA-approved as a collagenase inhibitor, and may be used between 3 and 9 months as an adjunctive therapy to periodontitis. The properties of doxycycline that make it an ideal SDD are that it is highly concentrated

in the gingival crevicular fluid (5–10 times greater than in serum), efficiently binds to tooth structures, demonstrates substantivity, and has the most potent anti-collagenase activity of the tetracycline family. The sub-antimicrobial dose of doxycycline in the dog is 1 mg/kg PO BID or 2 mg/kg PO once daily. Long-term administration doxycycline at a sub-antimicrobial dose has no reported antimicrobial resistance.

Answer 134 In veterinary dentistry, light-cured dental bonding agents are commonly used as an adhesive for composite restorations, or alone, for the purposes of dentin desensitization and sealing of patent dentin tubules. Secondary infection of the pulp through the ingress of bacteria through patent dentin tubules may occur, as in the case of acute uncomplicated crown fractures in young animals, and the application of a light-cured bonding agent to the dentin tubules may afford protection from infection. Specialized dentin desensitizing agents, such as Gluma® (Heraeus) may be used in combination with dental bonding agents. Dentin desensitizers act by penetrating into the dentin tubules, creating bridges that block fluid flow within the tubules.

Bonding agents bond to both etched enamel and to acid-treated dentin through micromechanical retention. In addition to the current sixth and seventh generation bonding agents, both fourth and fifth generation bonding agents, also referred to as total-etch adhesives, are still in use. Fourth and fifth generation bonding agents require a separate phosphoric acid etching step prior to application of the primer and adhesive, or single bottle combined primer and adhesive, and are typically associated with more postoperative sensitivity, especially if the dentin is over-dried following the etching phase. In contrast, the sixth and seventh generation bonding agents eliminate the phosphoric acid etching step all together, using an acid primer and adhesive or a single bottle acid primer and adhesive, are faster to apply, and have less reported postoperative sensitivity, but may have comparably weaker bonding strengths to enamel due to elimination of the phosphoric acid etching step. Bonding agents produce dentin bonding by using an initial hydrophilic agent which allows the resin to flow into the opened dentinal tubules. With fourth and fifth generation bonding agents, a comparatively thicker hybrid layer of resin and collagen forms the interface between the dentin and the overlying restoration. Over-drying the dentin collapses the collagen fibers, preventing a good bond, and also increases postoperative sensitivity. In comparison, sixth and seventh generation bonding agents directly incorporate the smear layer into the bonding substrate, which reduces sensitivity, but also results in a thinner hybrid layer. The hybrid layer – although not contributing significantly to the bond strength – acts as an efficient sealant preventing leakage of oral fluids and bacteria.

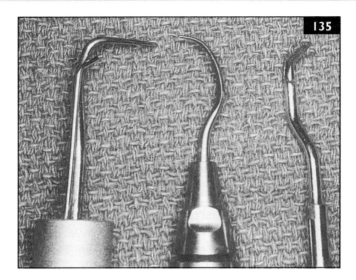

Question 135 Pictured are three different types of power scaling tips (**135**).
1 What are the different power sources for these instruments?
2 How does the tip action vary between these instruments, and what is their operating frequency?
3 What are the major similarities and differences of these power scalers?

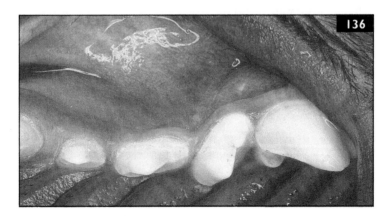

Question 136
1 What is abnormal about this dog's maxillary third premolar tooth (**136**), and what is the clinical significance of this condition?
2 How does this differ from deviation?

Answer 135

1 The scalers on the left and right are classified as ultrasonic scalers and are powered by electricity. The one on the left is a magnetostrictive unit. The electricity creates a magnetic field in a ferromagnetic rod or metal stack. This magnetic field creates vibrations which are transmitted to the working tip. The scaler on the right is classified as a piezoelectric unit. Electrical current is passed through a crystal in the handpiece that changes shape, thus creating the vibrations in the handpiece tip. The center scaler is a sonic scaler which is powered by compressed air and is attached to a dental handpiece. Vibrations at the scaler tip are created when air passes through a hole in a shaft inside the handpiece, spinning a ring which encircles the scaler.

2 The sonic scaler tip moves in an elliptical fashion, much like a figure-of-eight pattern. Sonic scalers operate at 2,000–6,000 Hz. The edges of the diamond-shaped tip are the most active and the power is concentrated in the last 3–5 mm of the tip. The ultrasonic tip on the left is equally active on all sides of the working end and moves in a rotary fashion. Pot-stack ultrasonic scaler tips have a more elliptical action or may have surfaces that are more active than others, namely the upper and under surfaces of the tip greater than the lateral surfaces. Ultrasonic scalers operate at frequencies of 20,000–40,000 Hz. Piezoelectric scalers have two active surfaces, usually the 3 o'clock and 9 o'clock sides. The tip motion is linear in a back-and-forth action. Piezoelectric scalers operate at 25,000–45,000 Hz. Knowledge of tip action and active sides of the instrument is important to allow for more efficient scaling and proper use of the instrument.

3 All these instruments are used for gross supragingival calculus removal from teeth. They all use a water spray for lavage and/or cooling and will create an aerosol. Different tip sizes and configurations are available for all of them for heavy calculus removal and fine calculus removal. The ultrasonic units will develop heat in the instrument tip, while the sonic scaler produces little heat. The ultrasonic magnetostrictive units with long and very thin tips with directed water spray are designed for subgingival use to perform periodontal débridement.

Answer 136

1 This tooth is rotated. Rotation refers to the movement of the tooth about its longitudinal axis. This is commonly seen in the upper third premolar teeth as a result of the overcrowding occurring in maxillary brachygnathia. In cases of malocclusion where the question arises whether the mandible is too long or the maxilla too short, this may be an indication of the latter. Rotation and crowding may also result in a distortion of the gingival contour, predisposing to plaque accumulation and periodontal disease.

2 Deviation (or *-version*) refers to the tilting of a tooth about its transverse axis. Persistent deciduous canine teeth may cause a lingual deviation (or *linguoversion*) of the mandibular permanent canine teeth, and a facial deviation (or *rostroversion*) of the maxillary permanent canine teeth.

Question 137 Masticatory muscle myositis (MMM) is an autoimmune, focal inflammatory myopathy limited to the muscles of mastication of the dog. Patients with MMM may present with exophthalmos, an acute swelling of the muscles of mastication and painful resistance to jaw opening, or in chronic cases, muscle atrophy-fibrosis and an inability to open the mouth (**137a**).

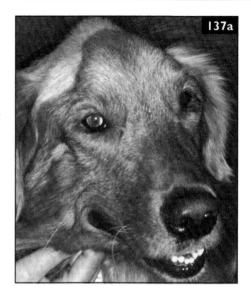

1 Name the muscles of mastication; which of these muscles are involved with MMM?
2 What tests are recommended for the diagnosis of MMM?
3 Which masticatory muscles are typically biopsied for the purposes of MMM, and what are the complications of biopsy?

Question 138 Mandibular drift associated with non-union mandibular fractures and following segmental mandibulectomy is a significant complication that results in difficulty prehending food, traumatic occlusion and injury to the contralateral temporomandibular joint. Discuss reconstructive techniques to prevent mandibular drift in patients with non-union mandibular fractures or following segmental mandibulectomy.

Question 139
1 Briefly describe the photoinitiated polymerization process of dental composites.
2 Describe the different types of dental curing lights.
3 Describe the function of this device (**139**).

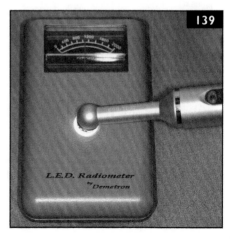

147

137–139: Answers

Answer 137

1 The masseter, temporal, and pterygoid (medial and lateral) muscles, muscles innervated by the mandibular branch of the trigeminal nerve, contain type 2M fibers, and are the masticatory muscles affected with MMM; whereas the digastricus muscle is comprised of type 2A fibers, and is not involved in the disease.

2 Serum creatine kinase (for the purposes of monitoring treatment), serum type 2M muscle antibody assay, muscle biopsy (immunohistochemical and histopathology), and CT. Although the serum test is highly sensitive and specific for MMM, false negatives are possible, especially in patients that have received or are receiving corticosteroid therapy for longer than 7–10 days, or in end-stage MMM patients where there is marked fibrosis and destruction of 2M fibers, and therefore the test should be combined with muscle biopsy for documentation of the degree of fibrosis and determination of prognosis. CT with contrast is a useful adjunctive test to aid in selection of sites for obtaining diagnostic biopsy samples; compared with the digastricus muscle, the temporal, masseter, and pterygoid muscles show inhomogeneous contrast enhancement (137b, arrows), and biopsies should ideally be obtained in the masticatory muscles with the most intense contrast enhancement. CT is also useful in ruling out other causes (e.g. disorders of the temporomandibular joint) for an inability to open the mouth.

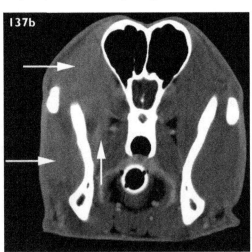

137b

3 The temporal and masseter muscles are the most accessible of the masticatory muscles for biopsy. Hemorrhage, incorrect biopsy of the superficial muscles (frontal and platysma), and iatrogenic trauma to the parotid salivary duct and local nerves are the most common complications seen with muscle biopsy. Ptosis and motor deficits of the cheek and lip may be seen if there is damage to the rostral auricular plexus and branches of the facial nerve, respectively.

Answer 138 Mandibular reconstruction to restore normal biomechanics and pain-free occlusion is the ideal treatment option to prevent mandibular drift. Reconstruction of critical-sized mandibular defects has traditionally been performed using a variety of techniques, including mandibular reconstruction plates, bone grafts, microvascular surgery and distraction osteogenesis, but these techniques are subject to limitations in graft size, failure of the grafts and morbidity associated with the donor sites. More recently, internal fixation techniques combined with regenerative biomaterials – bone morphogenetic proteins (BMPs) – have been described for the repair of non-union mandibular fractures and following segmental mandibulectomy. BMPs are a class of osteo-inductive growth factors capable of initiating the production of new bone. The challenge with the clinical use of BMPs has never been related to its ability to reliably form bone, but has been in finding an ideal volume and concentration of rhBMP-2 (i.e. clinically manufactured version of BMP), appropriate timing, and a suitable matrix to deliver the rhBMP-2 into the defect. Two veterinary case series have documented successful use of rhBMP-2 in the repair of non-union and segmental mandibular defects using internal fixation and a collagen sponge (MasterGraft® Matrix) cut to fit one-half to three-fourths the height of the bone defect and 2 mm greater than the defect length, infused with 50% of its volume with rhBMP-2 (**138a**). Use of this technique provided an immediate return to function and hard-tissue formation in as little as 2 weeks and cortical bone formation in 3 months (**138b**).

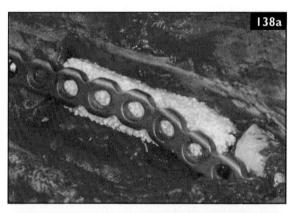

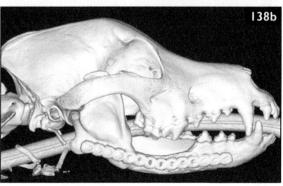

Answer 139

1 Camphorquinone (CPQ) is the most common photoinitiator used in dental composites. The major absorption wavelength of CPQ is 470 nm. The CPQ absorbs the photon energy of the light-curing unit and reacts with an amine activator that releases free radicals that initiate the polymerization reaction. Because CPQ is yellow in color, lighter shades of composite may use other photoinitiators that have an absorption wavelength below 400 nm. Therefore it is important to have a light-curing unit that can accommodate a wide range of wavelengths.

2 The two most common light technologies used today include quartz-tungsten halogen (QTH) and light-emitting diode (LED). QTH light-curing units typically run warm, are very energy inefficient, with only 10% of the total energy produced dedicated to light output and the other 90% to heat, and require a blue filter to produce light in the 450 to 500 nm range. Fans are necessary to cool QTH light-curing units, which are a hazard for aerosolization of bacteria from the patient. The bulbs themselves have a very limited lifespan, only 30 to 100 hours, before they begin to break down and need to be replaced. The filters of QTH units also degrade, crack, and discolor. Compared to traditional QTH units, LED curing units are cordless, energy efficient and durable. LED chips are long-lasting, and all later generation LED units are fine-tuned to the range of wavelengths used by all commonly used photoinitiators, including CPQ, phenyl-propanedione and Lucirin TPO, and are extremely efficient at utilizing every photon of energy produced for the light-curing process. Although the portability of cordless LED lights provides convenience, the batteries for these units may be a considerable expense to replace.

3 Radiometers are used to measure the light output (i.e. useful curing energy) of light-curing units in mW/cm² of light in the active range between 400 and 500 nm. There are no major differences between radiometers used for QTH bulbs and LED chips, and the same radiometer units may be used to measure the light output for both types of lights. Radiometers specifically calibrated for LED lights are available, however, and allow for high-output readings of up to 2,000 mW/cm². Although LED chips are durable and diodes may have a lifespan of up to 5,000 hours, their intensity may wane with prolonged use. Over time, material can build up on the light guides, the batteries of the unit may degrade, and careless handling/dropping of the unit may contribute to a reduction in light output. The light output of all curing lights, including LED lights, should be evaluated periodically with a radiometer to ensure thorough curing of dental materials.

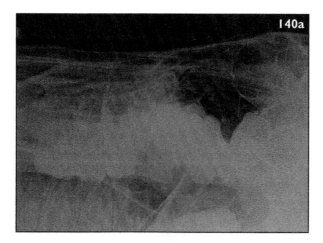

Question 140 A large swelling of the left maxilla was evident in this 9-year-old riding horse. Oral examination revealed a defect between the first and second molar teeth. Also shown here is a 30° lateral–oblique radiograph (140a).
1 What is the radiologic diagnosis?
2 How may the condition be treated?

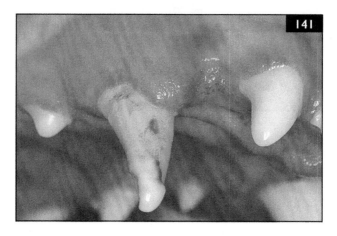

Question 141 The owner of this 1-year-old dog recalled that the deciduous precursor of this maxillary canine tooth (141) was fractured and extracted a few weeks later.
1 What is your diagnosis?
2 What are the therapeutic options?

140, 141: Answers

Answer 140

1 The radiograph shows a bizarre pattern of radiopaque tissues in the location of the first–third molar teeth, suggestive of an odontoma. An odontoma is an example of an inductive odontogenic tumor: during tumor formation, an inductive effect between the epithelial and mesenchymal tissues takes place, similar to that which occurs during odontogenesis, and the various dental tissues are formed. If tooth-like particles are identifiable, the term compound odontoma is used. In this case, where the aggregation of dental tissues is disorganized, this tumor is known as a complex odontoma. Although odontogenic tumors are rare in horses, the possibility of an odontogenic tumor should be considered whenever an animal develops a localized swelling, and particular suspicion should be raised when the patient is young, coinciding with the

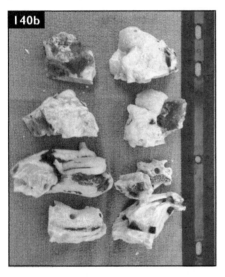

time of greatest activity of the primordial dental tissues. Although the radiologic signs of odontoma are pathognomonic, a biopsy is indicated in most cases.

2 An odontoma may be amenable to surgical removal. Removing the tumor by intracapsular excision (piecemeal withdrawal of the tumor) following a bone flap approach may be sufficient, but postoperative radiographs are advisable to establish that all dental tissue has been removed. In this case the tumor was removed via an oral approach utilizing minimal invasive buccotomy instruments (140b). Some odontomas are not amenable to surgical removal by virtue of their size.

Answer 141

1 Enamel hypoplasia is evident. The ameloblasts of the tooth germ of the permanent canine tooth were damaged during the first months of life, and subsequently no enamel was formed (see 75 and 127). There are two plausible explanations in this case. The fracture of the deciduous canine tooth may have been complicated (i.e. causing pulp exposure), with resultant pulp necrosis and periapical pathology. The periapical inflammation may have affected the underlying permanent tooth germ. Alternatively, the permanent tooth germ may have been damaged during the extraction of the deciduous tooth.

2 Given the fact that only one tooth is involved, restoration is indicated. A composite restoration using the acid-etch technique and a dentin-bonding agent will yield the most esthetic result. Alternatively, a metal-alloy jacket crown can be used.

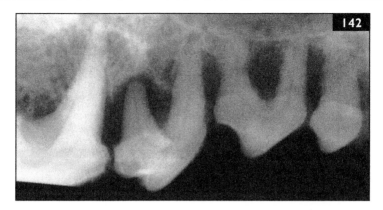

Question 142 This radiograph of a dog with periodontitis illustrates the radiologic findings typical of this disease process (142). Describe the radiographic features of periodontitis.

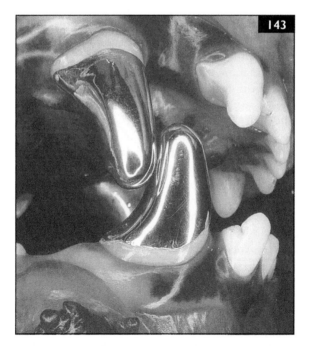

Question 143 A prosthetic crown is a restoration which replaces a part of the natural crown. What are the indications to perform a crown prosthesis in the dog (143)?

Answer 142 In advanced cases of periodontitis, the supporting bone peripheral to the lamina dura can appear either as more dense (sclerotic) or less dense (osteolysis) than healthy bone. The alveolar margin will often be lowered apically because of bony resorption. With horizontal bone loss the alveolar margin recedes parallel to the line connecting the cementoenamel junction; this can be seen affecting two or more adjacent teeth (**142**). Vertical bone loss (infrabony pockets) is seen involving single teeth or a single root of a tooth, and radiographically is either visualized as a wide periodontal space or as a 'cup' lesion of bone loss. Loss of bone attachment, advanced tooth mobility, gingival recession, and increased probing depths confirm periodontitis.

Radiographic assessment also reveals evidence of loss of marginal bone in the furcation area. This can be incomplete, known as furcation involvement (which clinically coincides with stage 1 or 2 furcation lesion) or complete, known as furcation exposure (which clinically coincides with a stage 3 furcation lesion). Periapical loss of bone is also evident leading to loss of attachment and tooth mobility. Reports state that approximately 40% of the bone must be demineralized before it can be detected radiographically.

Because of the unique patterns of periodontal bone loss associated with certain forms of periodontal disease, radiographs can provide useful diagnostic information. The main information provided by traditional radiography is an estimate of alveolar bone loss at the time of the radiographic survey. By comparing radiographs at different times, it is possible to estimate the loss or gain of bone at selected locations in the dentition.

Answer 143 The main indications for prosthetic crowns are fractured teeth or teeth with extensive abrasion. The dentition of domestic dogs (and cats) maintains its function even if parts of the dentition are missing or not functional. A crown fracture with pulp exposure requires endodontic treatment but prosthodontic build-up of the crown is optional. A prosthetic crown can also be used for the restoration of the normal gingival contour in crown-root fractures.

Fractured teeth should be restored if they are important to the normal function of a working dog. In working dogs, reduced crown height may lead to a diminished biting ability. A canine tooth that is shorter than normal, however, does not always cause problems in a working dog. If the remaining coronal portion of the tooth is healthy and long enough, and the dog is functioning well during training, crowning is not essential. However, there will always be a risk of repeated fracture of that canine tooth or fracture of one of the other canine teeth because the normal balance of the biting grip with four canine teeth has been lost.

Another indication for a prosthetic crown is to prevent further breakdown of the remaining tooth structure to prevent coronal fracture, for example: (1) in cage-biting dogs with worn canine teeth on the distal aspect (cage-biter syndrome); (2) in dogs with severely abraded teeth caused by destructive behavior like chewing on rocks or fences.

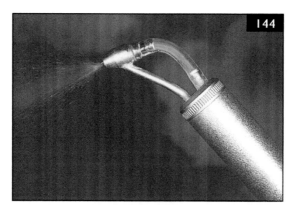

Question 144
1 This is the nozzle of a piece of equipment used during routine periodontal treatment (144). What is it, and how does it work?
2 What are the advantages of this technique?
3 How should it be used, and what precautions should be taken?

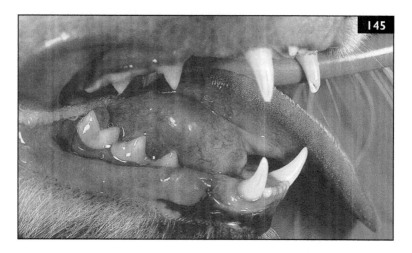

Question 145 This soft, fluid-filled, fluctuating swelling (145) is fairly typical for a condition commonly seen in the cat, but also in the dog.
1 Name and define this condition, and explain its pathogenesis.
2 What are the treatment options?

Answer 144

1 An air-polishing unit used for polishing. It uses medical-grade sodium bicarbonate crystals and water in a jet of compressed air to 'sandblast' the surface smooth. A well-known example of this equipment is the Prophy-Jet® (Dentsply Ltd.).

2 Air-polishing has many advantages, especially for veterinary use. It is a very effective means of polishing. Air-polishing involves no physical contact with the tooth and thermal injury is of no concern, contrary to cup-and-pumice polishing. Air-polishing is ideally suited for polishing teeth separated by wide interdental spaces and with a considerable variation in shape and size. Areas that are very difficult or even impossible to reach with the rubber cup can easily be polished using the air-polisher. It is also believed that air-polishing may be complementary to periodontal débridement in removing subgingival plaque and toxins.

3 The nozzle through which the slurry is propelled should be held 3–5 mm from the tooth and centered on the middle third of the tooth. The manufacturer's recommendation for conically shaped teeth is to direct the spray at a 60° angle towards the gingiva; however, care should be taken not to direct the spray directly into the sulcus. Non-keratinized mucosal surfaces (e.g. the sublingual mucosa) behind the teeth to be polished should be shielded, either by the operator's finger or by gauze. Prolonged use on dentin, cementum, and restorative materials (e.g. composite materials) should be avoided. There is some concern in human dentistry that absorption of the sodium bicarbonate may result in electrolyte disturbances. Air-polishing generates an aerosol of microorganisms and powder over a wide area around the patient. Personal protection (mask, eyewear) is, therefore, very important and work surfaces require thorough cleaning and disinfection after the procedure.

Answer 145

1 A *ranula* is a clinically descriptive term for a salivary mucocele that occurs specifically in the floor of the mouth and sublingually. Salivary mucoceles in the dog and cat are generally considered to be caused by extravasation of saliva, largely of unknown origin. Usually there is no history of trauma. Obstruction, simple transection of the duct, or trauma to glandular tissue does not cause a mucocele. Ligation of the duct causes atrophy of the gland involved. It is generally accepted that there is a lesion of the sublingual or mandibular salivary duct, or in one of the small ducts of the polystomatic sublingual salivary gland. Saliva leaks out and is not absorbed. This is irritating and causes the formation of a pseudocyst, lined by granulation tissue and macrophages. This pseudocyst is sometimes multilocular.

2 A ranula may be treated by intraoral marsupialization. An elliptical part of the ranula wall is excised. The edges are oversewn with a simple continuous suture, using thin synthetic absorbable suture material, to prevent premature closure.

Alternatively, or if the above procedure is unsuccessful, surgical excision of the monostomatic sublingual and mandibular salivary glands on the affected side is performed.

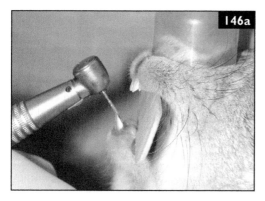
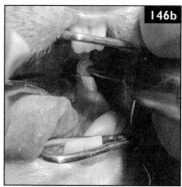

Question 146
1 How is occlusal adjustment and tooth-height reduction of incisor teeth (**146a**) in rabbits performed and what should be avoided?
2 How is occlusal adjustment and tooth-height reduction of premolar and molar teeth performed (**146b**)?

Question 147 This is a file in the access site for standard root canal treatment of a right maxillary canine tooth in a 4-year-old domestic shorthair cat (**147**).
1 Is it appropriate, in a case like this, where the crown of the maxillary canine tooth is fractured off at a point one-third from its cusp, to use the fracture site as the access site for standard root canal treatment?
2 Would you expect an easier and better access to the apex if the treatment access site were closer to the gingiva and on the mesial surface of this tooth?

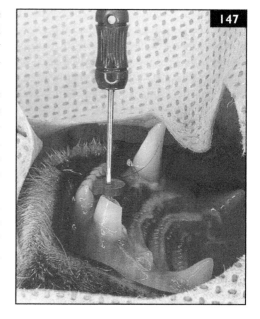

Answer 146

1 Tooth-height reduction of incisor teeth can be performed using a cylindrical diamond bur in a high-speed handpiece (**146a**). Care should be taken to avoid thermal damage to the pulp: a very light touch is used in order to avoid having to use cooling fluid; alternatively, the oropharynx can be packed, provided an endotracheal tube is used. A tongue depressor can be placed behind the incisor teeth to stabilize the jaws and protect the lips and tongue. Care should be taken to restore the normal occlusal plane angulation. If the tooth-height reduction is correctly performed, pulp exposure should not occur; however, if it does, a partial pulpectomy and direct pulp capping are indicated. An intermediate restorative material is used for filling the pulp cavity opening; harder materials like composites are not indicated, as they may interfere with normal attrition.

The use of a cutting disk on a surgical handpiece or Dremel™-tool is not recommended, as soft tissues are easily traumatized because of its size. Nail trimmers and wire cutters are contraindicated, as they crush the teeth, fracturing and splitting them, which in turn may cause pulp exposure. Not only is this very painful, but it may also lead to periapical pathology.

2 Occlusal adjustment of the premolar and molar teeth (**146b**), including height reduction and smoothing sharp points, can safely be performed using a round bur on a surgical handpiece. A cement spatula can be used for retracting and protecting the oral soft tissues. Small hand-held files are not very effective and tend to cause soft-tissue trauma. The bur can be dipped in cool saline or chlorhexidine solution to reduce the potential for thermal damage. Care should be taken to restore the normal occlusal plane angulation and to check the premolar–molar and incisor occlusion during the procedure. If one is not familiar with the normal anatomy and occlusion, it is advisable to have normal skull specimens available for reference.

Answer 147

1 In cats, the maxillary canine tooth is fairly straight. If the crown is fractured, access can be obtained at the fracture site. If the crown is intact, access can be made on the mesiobuccal aspect of the tooth, three-fourths of the distance from the gingival margin to the cusp. The more curved mandibular canine teeth of the cat should be approached in the same way as the mandibular canine teeth of dogs are approached, with access made 1–2 mm from the gingival margin on the mesial surface to the tooth.

2 The access would be more difficult if the site were closer to the gingiva in this case, as it would have to be more oblique. An obliquely directed access would result also in removing more tooth structure than desirable and in weakening this small tooth inappropriately.

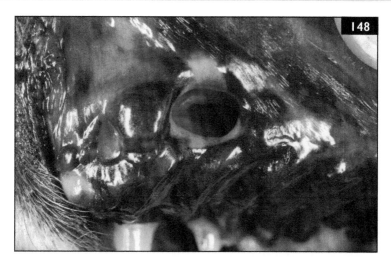

Question 148 This is an oral view of a 15-year-old miniature poodle, 3 weeks after the extraction of the left maxillary canine tooth (**148**). During the extraction of the tooth, a small amount of blood was evident at the left nostril.
1 What is your diagnosis, what is the most common cause of this condition, and where does it usually begin?
2 What general principles should be followed during the repair of this condition to ensure successful flap surgery? What are the indications for utilization of a single- versus a double-layer flap repair?

Question 149
1 What endodontic procedure is shown in this illustration (**149**)?
2 What are the indications for this procedure?
3 What are three types of filling materials that can be used in this procedure?

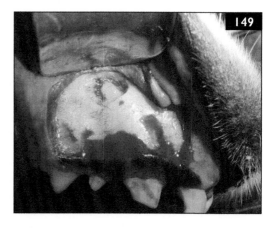

Answer 148

1 This is an acquired oronasal fistula, which is most commonly caused by periodontal disease. Periodontal disease that results in the development of an oronasal fistula most frequently begins on the palatal aspect of the maxillary canine tooth, when periodontal disease causes the destruction of the thin alveolar bone between the alveolus and the nasal cavity. Other teeth that can potentially be involved in oronasal fistula formation are the maxillary incisor teeth, the maxillary first and second premolar teeth, and the mesial root of the third premolar tooth. Fistula formation between the oral cavity and the maxillary recess may be associated with advanced periodontal disease of the distal root of the third premolar, fourth premolar, and first molar teeth.

2 General principles that should be followed to ensure successful oronasal repair surgery include the following: (1) The oronasal fistula should be débrided and the flap recipient site adequately prepared. (2) Flaps should be larger than the defects to be covered. (3) Flaps should be apposed without tension by releasing the periosteal layer and removing prominent buccal alveolar bone. (4) Tissues should be sutured to appose edges that do not have an intact epithelial surface. (5) Tissues should be gently handled. (6) A single-layer flap is usually sufficient for the repair of most recent oronasal fistulas. Recurrent or large fistulas may require the use of a double-layer flap.

Answer 149

1 A completed apicoectomy with a retrograde filling (surgical endodontic treatment).

2 A surgical endodontic procedure is indicated if there is failure of conventional root canal therapy associated with underfill or overfill of the root canal. Often, re-treatment with improved obturation will be sufficient to correct the problem and may be tried first. If there is evidence of persistent or increasing periapical changes radiographically after conventional root canal therapy with adequate obturation, an apicoectomy can be performed to remove the diseased root end and granulation tissue harboring persistent infection. Surgical endodontic therapy is often indicated if there are complications during conventional treatment, such as a separated instrument that precludes further treatment or a root end perforation that leads to failure. Additional indications for an apicoectomy would be if coronal access is impossible due to a stricture or calcified pulp chamber or if there is a horizontal fracture of the root tip.

3 The diseased apex is removed at an 80–90° angle to the long axis of the tooth. A cavity preparation is made using a bur on standard high-speed handpiece, or ultrasonically using special tips. The material of choice for the retrograde filling is MTA (Pro-Root, Dentsply). Other materials that can be used include a zinc oxide–eugenol intermediate restorative material (IRM™, Caulk) or a zinc oxide cement with alumina (Super EBA™, Bosworth).

Question 150 How would you classify the malocclusion of the right maxillary second molar tooth, seen on oral examination of this 10-year-old quarter horse gelding (**150**)?

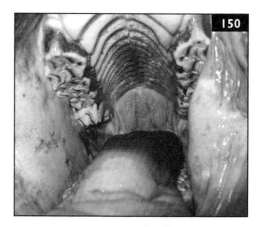

Question 151 Digital dental radiography is commonly used in veterinary dentistry (**151a, b**).
1 Discuss the different types of digital dental radiography commonly used in veterinary dentistry.
2 Which sizes of dental sensors, plates or film are recommended for veterinary dentistry?

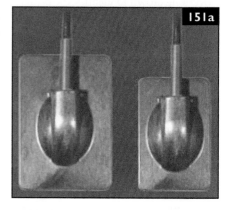

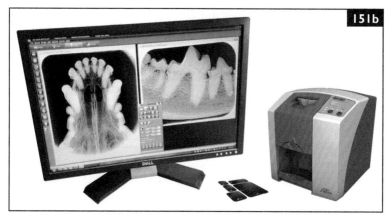

150, 151: Answers

Answer 150 When one tooth in the dental quadrants is causing a malocclusion it is considered a dental malocclusion. This is a class 1 malocclusion with one tooth causing the malocclusion.

In this case there is not a discrepancy in length of the maxilla to the mandible. This is evidenced by the lack of other malocclusions that are noted when the mandible occludes distal to the maxilla or vice versa. Malocclusions derived from a discrepancy in jaw lengths are considered skeletal malocclusions (class 2 or class 3). The overlong crown of the second molar tooth is a secondary response to lack of opposing dentition at the right mandibular second molar tooth. Whenever an overlong crown is identified, significant dental disease is often identified in the opposing quadrants to the overlong crown. Appropriate treatment would be occlusal adjustment with crown reduction in stages so as to not expose vital pulp of the second molar tooth. Occlusal thickness of dentin can vary but is on average 10–12 mm with older horses having less dentin. Examination of the dental quadrant opposing the overlong crown to identify the primary dental disease with imaging is warranted.

Answer 151

1 Direct digital imaging systems are commonly used in dental radiography. The majority of these systems are based on charge-coupled device (CCD) technology (**151a**). The disadvantages of CCD systems include the restrictions associated with the bulky sensor, connecting wire, limited sensor size (no size #4), and high sensor cost. Both wired (USB) or wireless sensors are available. Systems based on photo-stimulated phosphor (PSP) technology are also available (**151b**). Digital imaging based on PSP technology uses reusable imaging plates without cables or sensors, in combination with a conventional dental X-ray unit. The latent image is stored on the plate until processed by a laser scanner, and the image is displayed on the computer monitor. The plates are reusable and are relatively inexpensive. They are, however, sensitive to scratching, and this limits their lifespan. Processing of PSP plates does take almost as long as processing a full-set of conventional radiographs. They do offer the advantage of being available in size #4.

Digital radiography eliminates the costs and complications of film processing equipment, developer, fixer, cleaners, duplicating equipment, X-ray film, and mounts. Using these systems, radiation levels can be reduced by as much as 90%.

2 Five sizes of film are available (but not necessarily as sensors). Three of the sizes are commonly used in veterinary dental practice. Sizes #0 and #2 are known as periapical films, and size #4 as occlusal film.

Size	Dimensions (mm)	Possible use
#0	22 × 35	Mandibular P3-M1 in cats and very small dogs
#2	31 × 41	Standard size
#4	57 × 76	Occlusal views, large dogs

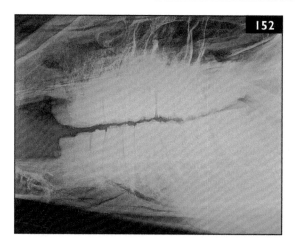

Question 152 An 18-year-old horse has sustained a traumatic injury to the left mandible. An acute swelling in the region with pain on palpation was noted, as well as mild dysphagia. A lateral radiograph (152) confirms a fracture which appears to involve the roots of the second, third and fourth premolar teeth. Suggest how this case should be managed.

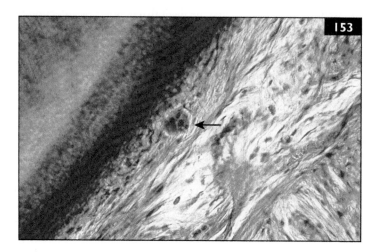

Question 153
1 What are the cells visible on this microphotograph (153, arrow) of the periodontal ligament of a dog?
2 What is the origin and clinical importance of these cells?
3 Where in the oral cavity can similar cells be found, and what are they called?

Answer 152 Fracture of the body of the mandible should always be considered in cases of acute swelling of the jaw. External palpation, intraoral examination, and a careful radiographic investigation are used for diagnosis. The principles that relate to the treatment of facial trauma are no different to those which apply to other wounds: control of hemorrhage and preservation of vital functions such as respiration in the acute phase; anatomic restoration and restoration of normal dental occlusion; removal of devitalized tissue; and control of secondary infection. It is rare for facial wounds to be so severe that surgery is required to stop hemorrhage and to maintain patent nasal airways. Open wounds over the sinuses may necessitate removal of loose bone fragments and débridement of gross contamination. An implanted irrigation catheter can be a useful measure to flush away blood and debris and should always be used when the sinus wall has sustained a full-thickness penetration. The provision of broad-spectrum antibiotic cover during the immediate post-traumatic period should be routine. Most bone fragments retain periosteal or endosteal attachments and heal uneventfully, but occasionally devitalization leads to sequestration with a discharge to the nose or skin surface. These should be dealt with by surgical removal as and when they arise. Grossly deforming depression fractures should be treated by elevation as soon as possible after the trauma; otherwise a fibrous union will form in a matter of days. Many fractures of the mandible show little displacement of the bone fragments and surgical fixation is often not necessary. Dietary alteration to a soft diet to reduce the need for mastication is advised. However, teeth may be devitalized either by infection through the fracture line or by disruption of their vascular supply. The decision whether or not to extract depends on radiographic findings, but this should be delayed at least until a firm fibrous union of the fracture site is present. Attempts to extract before this time may exacerbate any displacement of the mandibular fragments.

Answer 153
1 These clusters of epithelial cells are known as the epithelial cell rests of Malassez.
2 They are remnants of Hertwig's epithelial root sheath. The double layer of epithelial cells of this sheath grows around the dental papilla. The cells initiate the differentiation of odontoblasts on the periphery of the dental papilla and the odontoblasts in turn form the dentin of the root. As the root is formed, the sheath is stretched and fragments. In erupted teeth some of these epithelial cells persist next to the root surface within the periodontal ligament. The epithelial cells of Malassez play a role in the histogenesis of the periapical cyst, lateral periodontal cyst, and (intraosseous) ameloblastoma. Their role in the repair and maintenance of the periodontal ligament is unclear, but probably minimal.
3 Remnants of the dental lamina are occasionally seen in the dense connective tissue of the gingiva as clusters of epithelial cells, known as the cell rests of Serres. It is thought that these cell rests may be involved in the pathogenesis of canine acanthomatous ameloblastoma.

Question 154 A 2-year-old, castrated male terrier was presented for evaluation of a 2-week history of ptyalism, gagging, and bilateral mandibular salivary gland enlargement. Histopathology of the mandibular salivary glands, routine laboratory testing (CBC, serum chemistry, and urinalysis), and thoracic radiographs were unremarkable.

1 Name the major salivary glands in the dog. How common is salivary gland disease, what is the most common salivary gland condition, and what is the most likely diagnosis in this case?

2 What is the recommended treatment/management of this condition?

Question 155 Aging and pathologic effects, such as attrition, abrasion, erosion, uncomplicated fractures, and caries, elicit a reaction of the dentin–pulp complex.

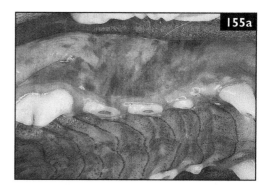

1 Define the terms abrasion and attrition.

2 Describe the defense mechanism of the dentin to wear of dental hard tissue.

3 In cases of attrition or abrasion, the central area of the incisal or occlusal surface of the tooth may have a dark color, as seen in this example of abrasion caused by chewing tennis balls (**155a**). How can this be differentiated from caries or the exposed pulp of a complicated crown fracture?

Question 156 A post-and-core build-up and prosthetic crown were used in this case (**156a**).

1 What does this technique involve, and what is it used for?

2 Describe the procedure used.

3 What are the potential complications?

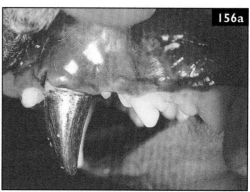

Answer 154
1 The four major salivary glands in the dog are the mandibular, zygomatic, parotid, and sublingual glands (154). Diseases of the salivary glands are uncommon, and include sialocele, sialolithiasis, sialadenitis/necrotizing sialometaplasia (salivary infarction)/sialodenosis (sialosis) and neoplasia (adenocarcinoma). The zygomatic glands are the least affected by disease. Sialoceles are regarded as the most common disease of the salivary glands. In this case, based upon the clinical presentation and benign histopathology of the mandibular salivary gland, the diagnosis, by exclusion, is most consistent with sialodenosis. Patients with sialodenosis of the mandibular glands usually present with retching and vomiting clinical signs, and the diagnosis of sialodenosis is typically one of exclusion, but may occur concurrently with other salivary gland conditions (e.g. sialocele). The markedly enlarged mandibular salivary glands are non-painful, but may evoke gagging, coughing or vomiting symptoms when palpated. In the case of sialodenosis, fine-needle aspiration cytology and/or incisional biopsy are unremarkable. Dogs with sialadenitis and necrotizing sialometaplasia of the mandibular glands often are presented with similar clinical signs, but differ in their histopathology and are painful to palpation of the enlarged glands.

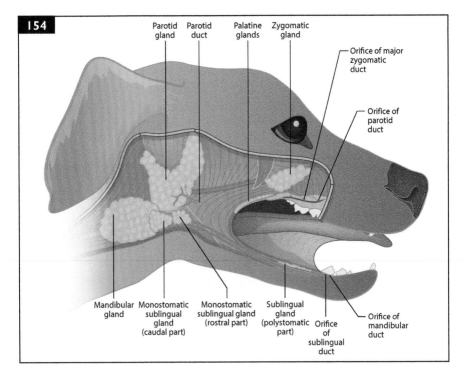

154

Parotid gland | Parotid duct | Palatine glands | Zygomatic gland

Orifice of major zygomatic duct

Orifice of parotid duct

Mandibular gland | Monostomatic sublingual gland (caudal part) | Monostomatic sublingual gland (rostral part) | Sublingual gland (polystomatic part) | Orifice of sublingual duct | Orifice of mandibular duct

2 Sialodenosis may be a form of limbic (or temporal lobe) epilepsy (i.e. seizures that manifest as behavioral changes), and is classically treated using phenobarbital or other anti-convulsants (potassium bromide or levetiracetam – Keppra®). Response to treatment is usually quick, 24–48 hours, and may be tapered off over the course of 6 months; however, in some cases, life-long therapy is necessary to prevent recurrence.

Answer 155

1 Attrition and abrasion are terms that are often confused. Attrition is a physiologic process that can be defined as a gradual and regular loss of tooth substance (wear) as result of natural mastication. If attrition is caused by abnormal function or malocclusion, the excessive wear caused by tooth-to-tooth contact is called pathologic attrition. Abrasion refers to mechanical wear other than by normal mastication or tooth-to-tooth contact, e.g. wear caused by chewing rocks, bars, or wire.

2 The primary dentin includes the first layers of dentin formed during odontogenesis. Under normal conditions, formation of dentin continues throughout life and secondary dentin is deposited on the entire pulpal surface of the primary dentin. Extensive wear exposes the odontoblastic processes of the odontoblasts and these cells may degenerate as a result of this wear. However, it is more common for these cells to survive the traumatic insult and to be stimulated to form the reactionary tertiary dentin. Tertiary dentin has a less organized structure than primary and secondary dentin and stains easily. This is evidenced as a brown area in the middle of the incisal or occlusal surface. At times, the teeth may be worn to the gingival margin without exposure of the dental pulp. This is possible because the pulp responds with a progressive formation of tertiary dentin.

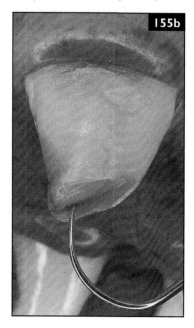

155b

3 A fresh exposure of vital pulp will bleed and cause acute pain when probed with a dental explorer. If left untreated, the opening in the pulp chamber with the exposed pulp stays open and becomes brown or black in appearance and occluded with necrotic material. However, it always remains possible to introduce a dental explorer into the pulp chamber, as shown this photograph (155b). In case of attrition or abrasion the colored central area is hard with no pulp exposure. An early carious lesion usually appears brown or black and will feel slightly soft or 'sticky' when probed

with a fine dental explorer. A carious cavity involving the dentin is filled with disintegrated dental substance and debris. The walls of the cavity are lined with contaminated decalcified dentin, in contrast to resorption defects, which are lined by healthy, hard dental substance.

Answer 156

1 There are two types of post-and-core build-ups. The first type is the use of a post in the pulp chamber/root canal and build-up of a restorative material around the post before a crown preparation, as in **156b**. The second type is the shaping of the pulp chamber and subsequent creation by a dental laboratory of a custom post-and-core with a crown to fit over the post-and-core. A post-and-core technique is used to lengthen the crown height when the remaining natural tooth does not have enough height for the placement of a prosthetic crown.

2 First, endodontic therapy is performed. In the first type, an endodontic post or dowel is selected that is slightly less than one-third the width of the tooth. A Peeso-reamer of corresponding size or, in some cases, a bur is used to open the canal and remove the gutta-percha down to the desired depth. It is important to make as clean a cut into the tooth as possible. Wobble of the reamer may cause a non-circular canal and prevent a tight fit of the post. A trial fit of the dowel is made. The dowel is cemented in place with a glass-ionomer or resin cement. A small pin may be placed parallel to the post to increase stability. A composite resin is placed over the post to build up the crown. A routine crown preparation is performed. In the custom post-and-core technique, the pulp chamber is prepared with a 5–10° wall preparation. A routine crown preparation is performed. Impression material is first inserted into the pulp chamber and then around the remaining crown and adjacent gingiva. To strengthen the post impression, a needle, toothpick, small wire, or other object may be inserted into the pulp chamber before inserting the impression material; or, these stiffeners may be inserted just after inserting the impression material but before coating the crown with the impression material.

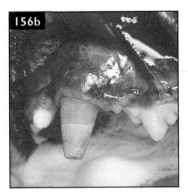

3 The greatest complication of this type of treatment is subsequent fracture of the tooth due to the external stresses that may cause fracture of the supporting walls of tooth. To overcome this, the ratio of the exposed length should be at least one length of exposed post to one to two lengths of post depth. For example, if the desired height of post build-up is 10 mm, the post depth should be 10–20 mm. This added length of the post helps to distribute the forces down the root.

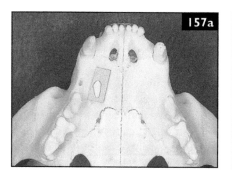
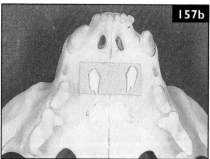
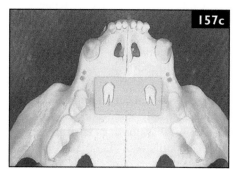

Question 157 What is the anatomic–zoological importance of the small teeth shown (**157a–c**)?

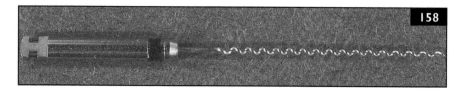

Question 158 This is a Lentulo® paste filler (**158**).
1 How is it used?
2 What are its advantages?
3 What are its disadvantages?

Answer 157 The most mesial maxillary premolar tooth in the cat is the second premolar tooth. The normal dental formula of the cat is identical with that of virtually all other members of the Family Felidae, Subfamily Felinae, namely:

$$I\frac{3}{3}:C\frac{1}{1}:P\frac{3}{2}:M\frac{1}{1}=30$$

The maxillary second premolar tooth has received considerable attention from zoologists, its absence being interpreted as indicating a tendency towards reduced dentition in the cat, as compared with the original carnivore dentition. The maxillary second premolar tooth was found to be absent in 3.4–28.4% of cat populations worldwide, and it was postulated that the tendency towards absence of the maxillary second premolar tooth increased from North to South. The tooth is also frequently absent in the cheetah (*Acinonyx jubatus*), caracal (*Caracal caracal*), manul (*Otocolobus manul*), leopard cat (*Prionailurus bengalensis*), lynx (*Lynx lynx*) and bobcat (*L. rufus*). The tooth varies considerably in size and position. The maxillary second premolar tooth is generally described as a single-rooted tooth, although two (often fused) roots occur. In one study, 20% of maxillary second premolar teeth present had partly fused double roots, while 2% had two fully formed roots. This is of clinical importance if extraction of this tooth is indicated.

Illustrated are three cat skulls with (**157a**) unilateral absence of left maxillary second premolar tooth and a normally shaped right maxillary second premolar tooth; (**157b**) bilaterally present maxillary second premolar teeth with partly fused double roots; and (**157c**) bilaterally present maxillary second premolar teeth with fully formed double roots.

Answer 158

1 Paste fillers are used with a slow-speed handpiece and a reduction contra-angle to deliver root canal sealers to the apical third of the root canal at the beginning of the obturation stage of standard root canal therapy. The instrument is inserted, loaded with sealer, to the apical portion of the canal, and rotated as it is withdrawn from the canal. The twist of the paste filler is in a counterclockwise direction and it unloads the sealer as the instrument is withdrawn, being rotated clockwise.

2 The primary advantage of using a paste filler is in obtaining a uniform coating of sealer at the apical end of the canal and on the canal walls, ensuring that the open dentinal tubules will be sealed when gutta-percha is vertically or laterally condensed in the canal.

3 The instrument must be used at a speed not exceeding 5,000 rpm, utilizing a reduction-gear contra-angle, and it will break easily if stressed. Stress will be applied to the paste filler when it is rotated within a curved canal, or if it is inserted in a canal that is too narrow.

Question 159 This is a picture of the palatal surface of the left maxillary fourth premolar tooth (159) in a 12-year-old pit bull dog; it is representative of the general appearance of all the premolar and molar teeth. In addition to a professional dental cleaning, the dog was presented for evaluation and treatment of multiple fractured teeth. Describe the condition present on the crown of this tooth. What are potential causes of this condition? Is treatment indicated?

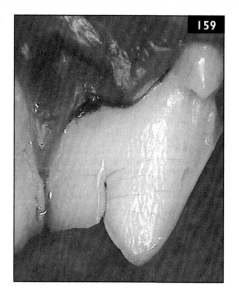

Question 160 A young adult female standard poodle is presented for treatment of a fractured canine tooth with pulp exposure; the fracture occurred while the dog was boarding at a local kennel. The owners are concerned that the tooth is painful. The dog has had a poor appetite and has been lethargic since they brought her home the previous evening. She vomited a yellow liquid this morning; this is not unusual for her after she has been boarded at a kennel. Physical examination was unremarkable except for the fractured tooth and dehydration estimated at 5%. Preanesthesia blood work findings included:

BUN 63.9 mmol/l (urea 90 mg/dl) (normal 4.3–21.3 mmol/l; urea 6–30 mg/dl))
Creatinine 265 mmol/l (3.0 mg/dl) (normal 62–115 mmol/l; 0.7–1.3 mg/dl)
Sodium 132 mmol/l (normal 145–155 mmol/l)
Chloride 98 mmol/l (normal 104–117 mmol/l)
Potassium 7.0 mmol/l (normal 4.0–5.4 mmol/l)
Total calcium 13.0 mg/dl (normal 9.8–12.8 mg/dl)
Albumin 35 g/l (normal 26–36 g/l)
Urine specific gravity 1.020

1 What is your assessment of these laboratory data?
2 What other laboratory tests are indicated?

159, 160: Answers

Answer 159 This is enamel infraction, which is a crack or incomplete fracture (craze line) of the crown substance confined to the enamel. There is no loss of tooth structure with infraction; the enamel is fractured but remains adherent to the underlying dentin. Primary radiographic changes are not associated with the condition, but evaluation for secondary traumatic injury to the roots, luxation, loss of vitality or periapical pathosis is warranted. Infraction is most commonly observed in older patients from accumulated dental trauma or iatrogenic injury from dental instruments. The prognosis for infracted teeth is uneventful, and treatment, if performed, would be for cosmetic reasons only; a light-cured resin may be applied to the affected areas to prevent discoloration of the craze lines (i.e. that may occur if the craze lines propagate allowing organic debris to fill into the cracks).

Answer 160
1 The extent of blood testing before anesthesia is dependent upon physical examination findings, historical information, preventive health care provided (e.g. heartworm prevention), and the patient's age. Lethargy and reluctance to eat are non-specific clinical signs which may result from oral disease and pain or many other diseases. Patients that have systemic signs of disease, as does this patient, should have a minimum laboratory database to include a complete blood count (CBC), renal function tests, electrolytes, liver enzymes, and urinalysis. Anesthesia and treatment of the fractured tooth should be delayed until the patient has been managed medically and is stable for anesthesia.

The abnormalities identified in this patient include azotemia, hyponatremia, hypochloridemia, hyperkalemia, and hypercalcemia. Based on the history and laboratory results, hypoadrenocorticism should be high on the differential diagnosis list; this is a common disease in young adult standard poodles, with females being affected twice as often than males. Differential diagnoses for azotemia are prerenal, renal, and/or postrenal in origin. Postrenal azotemia may be ruled out based on history and physical examination. The urine specific gravity may be helpful in differentiating renal from prerenal causes of azotemia. The urine specific gravity indicates abnormal concentrating ability in this patient; however, the ability to concentrate urine is altered in patients with hypoadrenocorticism. Hypoadrenocorticism may cause decreased renal medullary sodium concentration and therefore a decreased ability to concentrate urine. Prerenal azotemia is commonly associated with hypoadrenocorticism and should resolve with appropriate fluid therapy. Patients in which the azotemia does not resolve with appropriate fluid therapy may have concurrent acute or chronic renal damage.
2 A CBC was performed in this patient and the lack of a stress response was consistent with a patient with hypoadrenocorticism. An ACTH-stimulation test is recommended to confirm a diagnosis of hypoadrenocorticism; if the diagnosis is confirmed preoperative supplementation of corticosteroids is recommended.

Question 161 This is the buccal view of a dog presented because of discomfort during eating (161). The owner also reports that blood is sometimes seen mixed with drooled saliva. What next steps are indicated in order to obtain a diagnosis for this dog?

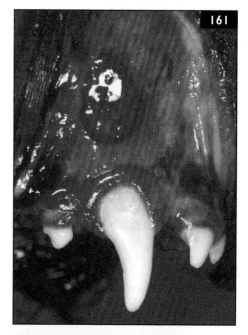

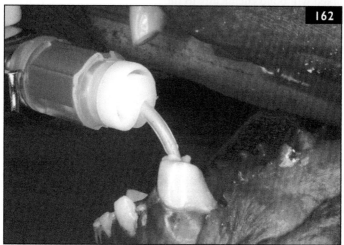

Question 162 Obturation of the root canal has been completed and the walls of the access site have been prepared. Which intermediate restorative material is being applied (162) for restoration of the access site of this root canal treatment, and why?

Answer 161 The affected areas seen are those associated with contact mucositis and contact mucosal ulceration. These lesions are often referred to as 'contact ulcers' or 'kissing ulcers', and are seen on areas of the oral mucosa or lateral edge of the tongue where the tissues are in contact with the plaque-laden surfaces of teeth.

A thorough oral and physical examination and history are very important first steps in diagnosis. Rule in or out: systemic infection; autoimmune diseases (mucocutaneous junction lesions, or lesions generalized in the mouth, including the hard palate); cold agglutinin disease (lesions of the edges of the tongue or lips, and tips of the tail or ears); epidermal necrolysis secondary to administration of medications; access to toxins; abnormal chewing habits; and neoplasia. Breed can be important: Maltese dogs are the classic breed affected by ulcerative stomatitis, and cavalier King Charles spaniels develop eosinophilic pharyngeal ulcers. Biopsy is indicated to differentiate contact mucositis from autoimmune disease and other conditions, including neoplasia. Bacterial culture is difficult to interpret because of the presence of the multibacterial oral flora.

Answer 162 A tooth-colored glass-ionomer restorative would be an ideal selection as intermediate restorative material for the access site of this root canal treatment. Glass-ionomers are a combination of glass and polyacrylic acid that when mixed will bond chemically to the tooth in an acid–base reaction that does not require an adhesive. Compared to composites, glass-ionomers are less hydrophobic, more tolerant of any residual moisture that the operator cannot see, and the acid–base reaction actually requires water; therefore, the preparation of the site only needs to be reasonably dry. The resultant chemical bond to the tooth is very strong, resistant to microleakage, and is not predisposed to shrinkage as are composites that cure via a polymerization reaction. Glass-ionomers have a coefficient of expansion similar to dentin, and they are generally considered to be a good dentin replacement. Another benefit of the glass-ionomer class of materials is the continuous release of fluoride, which in humans is particularly beneficial in reducing secondary caries. As a class of restorative materials, however, glass-ionomers have poor wear resistance and strength, making them sufficient for use as an intermediate restorative material in a 'sandwich' technique between the final composite restoration, but not as the sole access site restoration unless intended as a temporary restoration of the access site. An example of the latter would be when a root canal treatment is staged between the cleaning/shaping phase and the final canal obturation phase of the treatment. Glass-ionomer restorations also lack translucency, stain resistance, and are not as esthetic as composites. Resin-modified glass-ionomers include a resin polymer that will polymerize when light cured; this improves on the strength and esthetics of the restorative material, but its abrasion and wear characteristics are still lacking.

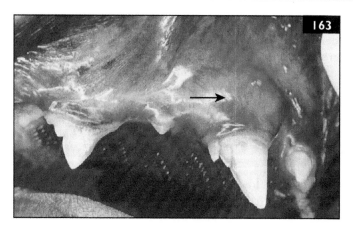

Question 163 This 6-year-old domestic shorthair cat was presented for examination (**163**). The right maxillary canine tooth crown is fractured and there is also a small draining tract visible over the root area (arrow).
1 What are two possible causes of the draining tract in this case?
2 What locations of this sinus tract will give you a clue as to the source of the opening?
3 What additional steps can be taken to confirm your diagnosis?

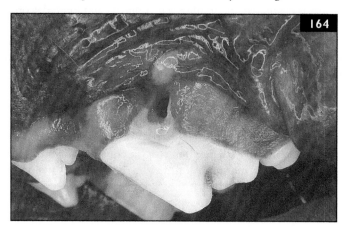

Question 164
1 Name the lesion on the fourth premolar tooth (**164**), and describe a method of characterizing its severity.
2 What is the prognostic significance of this lesion?
3 What are the therapeutic options?

Answer 163

1 (1) Endodontic disease associated with the exposed pulp secondary to the complicated crown fracture. (2) Periodontitis.

In this case the draining tract developed secondary to periodontal disease associated with a crown–root fracture with a loose root fragment.

2 A draining tract coronal to the mucogingival line is typically associated with periodontal disease. If the opening of the draining tract is at or apical to the mucogingival line, it is known as a 'parulis' and there is endodontic disease with a periapical abscess.

3 When an oral draining tract is detected, a periodontal probe is used to check for periodontal attachment loss and an intraoral radiograph is obtained. A gutta-percha point may be placed into the draining tract to assist in locating the source of the tract.

Answer 164

1 A furcation lesion which represents bone resorption between the roots of multirooted teeth. The severity of furcation lesions can be classified: *Stage 1*: the division between the roots can be felt with a probe but is less than 3 mm deep. *Stage 2*: a probe can pass horizontally into the furcation for more than 3 mm but not all the way through. *Stage 3*: a probe can be passed all the way through the furcation to the opposite aspect of the tooth (e.g. buccal to lingual on a maxillary second premolar tooth in a dog). Ideally, in charting, each aspect of the division between roots is evaluated and graded, e.g. a buccal and lingual score is given for the furcation area of the mandibular first molar tooth of the dog.

2 This lesion indicates the presence of chronic, advanced periodontitis. Generally, the presence of furcation lesions significantly worsens the prognosis for long-term retention of teeth despite therapy because it is more difficult to clean such areas as they are prone to retain food debris and plaque.

3 Two procedures have been advocated to eliminate furcation exposure: hemi-section and guided tissue regeneration. The latter procedure is currently the most popular but is limited to stage 2 furcations at the present time. This procedure consists of a flap approach with maximum tissue conservation by making incisions very close to the gingival margin. A full-thickness flap is elevated taking care not to tear or damage the vascularity of the flap. Flap vitality is critical because flap necrosis usually results in failure to regenerate the furcation. The bony margins of the defect are exposed by curettage and all soft-tissue tags are removed in order to prevent soft tissue from filling in the healing wound. The roots are cleaned and smoothed so that irregularities do not interfere with flap or membrane adaptation to the tooth. A barrier membrane is adapted to the tooth and over the bony walls of the furcation defect in such a way as to create space for bone growth and occlude overlying soft tissue from the defect during healing. The soft tissue is closed over the defect and well adapted to the tooth so that fibrin or a blood clot can seal the furcation defect away from oral bacteria.

Question 165 This photograph (165a) shows the normal incisor tooth occlusion in an adult, standard-sized rabbit. The tips of the chisel-shaped mandibular incisor teeth occlude between the maxillary first and second incisor teeth when the jaw is relaxed. The breeding of animals to alter their appearance frequently has a detrimental effect on the function of the affected anatomic structures. As with dogs which have

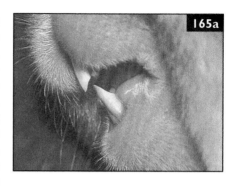

been bred for a short muzzle and 'flat' face, rabbit breeds with this tendency suffer from increased respiratory problems and jaw length mismatch.

1 What is the main structural change in the head of dwarf breed rabbits when compared with their naturally occurring wild counterparts?
2 At what age are dwarf rabbits with incisor tooth malocclusion usually presented to the veterinarian, and why?
3 Several treatment options are available for rabbits with incisor tooth malocclusion as a result of jaw length mismatch. Briefly what are they?

Question 166 Dental plaque (166) is made of bacteria.
1 What is the sequence of events leading to the formation of dental plaque?
2 Is dental plaque unique?
3 What is the bacterial composition of plaque, and how does it change with disease?

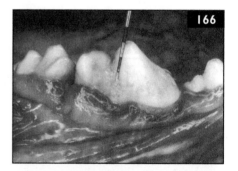

Question 167 Tooth brushing is the single most effective means of removing plaque (167).
1 What frequency of tooth brushing is required to maintain clinically healthy gingiva?
2 Which toothbrush and tooth brushing technique is recommended?

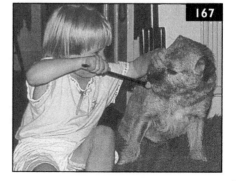

Answer 165

1 The dwarf breeds of rabbit have a shorter head than normal. The main area affected is the base of the skull. This affects the length of the upper jaw and location of the temporomandibular joints. Although the mandible is usually reduced in length, the degree of shortening is often insufficient so that there is a relative mandibular prognathism.

2 A high proportion of dwarf rabbits have relative mandibular prognathism with malocclusion of the incisor teeth. This may be observed in newborn rabbits, but most cases are presented at between 9 and 18 months of age. A case of incisor tooth malocclusion in a 3-month-old dwarf rabbit with relative mandibular prognathism is shown (165b). This condition was not visible until the lips were lifted. It frequently takes 9–18 months for the incisor teeth to wear in

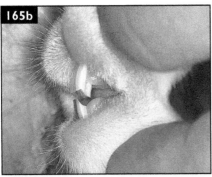

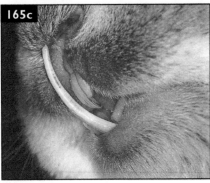

such a way that they no longer occlude with the opposing teeth. As the teeth can then grow unimpeded, it is not long before the teeth become visibly elongated. This is the most common reason for owners to present affected animals. The second most frequent reason is loss of weight or condition. This was the case in this 13-month-old dwarf rabbit (165c). The owners were not aware that the visible elongation of the mandibular incisor teeth was abnormal and they had not noticed that the tips of these teeth were penetrating the nasal skin. This abnormality drastically restricts the ability of affected animals to prehend and chew food.

3 The most frequent treatment used in cases such as those described in (2) is regular occlusal adjustment. Extraction of the incisor teeth is another treatment option.

Answer 166

1 The oral cavity is colonized by bacteria soon after birth. After tooth eruption, the tooth surface and the gingival sulcus constitute new ecological niches. The tooth surface is covered by an acellular organic film of salivary proteins

and glycoproteins. These are adsorbed onto the hydroxyapatite of the tooth surface to form the dental pellicle. Initial plaque formation begins with attachment of bacteria via physical forces on the pellicle (association of bacteria). Not all bacteria are able to attach to the tooth surface. Initial colonization in humans is due to specific bacteria (*Streptococcus sanguis*, *Actinomyces* sp.) that can both attach to the tooth surface and provide attachment to other bacteria via receptors. Multiplication of attached bacteria and adhesion of new bacteria provide initial growth. Coaggregation reactions between initial bacteria and other bacteria (that are unable to attach to tooth surfaces) provide further growth of the dental plaque, forming a highly organized self-sustaining community of several hundred species of bacteria, the biofilm.

2 Communities within plaque develop depending on the site and time of development. There is not one dental plaque but different dental plaques that differ according to their ecological niche (smooth surface, pits and fissures, gingival sulcus, periodontal pocket, etc.). Virulence properties of specific plaque inhabitants are well defined. *Streptococcus mutans*, which ferments dietary carbohydrate to form lactic acid, is responsible for caries in humans and represents only 1% of the salivary flora; it is not a predominant bacteria in supra- or subgingival plaque, but represents 25% of the flora in an occlusal fissure. On the contrary, *Porphyromonas gingivalis*, which is associated with severe periodontal disease in humans, is mostly found in deep periodontal pockets. Physicochemical conditions on the tooth surface and in the gingival sulcus or in the periodontal pocket are not the same; subsequently, supragingival plaque and subgingival plaque differ.

3 Dental plaque is composed of aerobic, facultative, and anaerobic species. In humans, plaque initially comprises predominantly oral *Streptococci* and *Actinomyces*. With the development and worsening of periodontal disease, subgingival plaque composition changes from aerobic, Gram-positive, non-motile species to predominantly anaerobic, motile, Gram-negative species. With periodontitis, anaerobes represent 80–90% of subgingival plaque. Most knowledge on bacterial composition of plaque and biofilm formation process is obtained from human medicine, as data on animals are rare, but the oral microflora in animals differ significantly, especially at the genus and species level. For example, only 16.4% of oral taxa are shared between dogs and humans. Also, most recent studies show that healthy canine plaque lacks *Streptococci* and is dominated by Gram-negative bacterial species, where Gram-positive anaerobic species prevail in disease. In dogs, the most predominant phyla of the oral flora in general are *Bacteroidetes*, *Proteobacteria*, *Firmicutes* and *Actinobacteria*. The shift in the proportion of these bacteria occurs between health (most abundant *Proteobacteria* and *Bacteroidetes*) and disease (mild periodontitis), where *Firmicutes* prevail in the microflora. Most commonly recognized bacteria associated with periodontal disease in

dogs include *Actinomyces*, *Peptostreptococcaceae* and *Porphyromonas* spp., and less commonly *Treponema denticola*.

Answer 167

1 One study has shown that brushing every other day is sufficient to maintain clinically healthy gingiva in the dog. Another study failed to duplicate these results. More recently, a 28-day randomized, controlled and blinded study in laboratory beagle dogs confirmed that daily tooth brushing produced a statistically significant reduction in plaque (37%), calculus (80%) and existing gingivitis (60%) compared to non-brushed control dogs. A significant reduction in plaque (25%), calculus (65%) and gingivitis (41%) was also identified for every-other-day tooth brushing compared with non-brushed control dogs. No significant recorded difference in plaque reduction was seen with tooth brushing once weekly or once every other week compared to non-brushed control dogs. Consequently, dog owners should be instructed to provide tooth brushing daily, or no less frequently than every other day, to achieve a significant retardation in plaque and calculus, and reduction in gingivitis.

2 A toothbrush compliant with the American Dental Association standard ISO 20126:2005 was used in dogs in a trial conducted according to Veterinary Oral Health Council (VOHC) protocols. A child-sized brush with soft bristles and a flat profile head was used. The bristles have rounded tips to avoid damaging the gingiva. Brushes that meet this standard are marketed by several manufacturers.

The brush is to be applied to the surfaces of the teeth at a 45° angle, with the tips of the bristles pointed towards the gingival tissue. The brush is pressed gently against the buccal surface of the tooth during the brush stoke – if the bristles visibly deflect (curve), the pressure applied is too high. Three horizontal strokes, each consisting of a back-and-forth movement, are made, covering a specific 'set' of several teeth at a time in each stroke, and a fourth stroke is made, directing the brush away from the gingiva towards the tip of the crowns of the teeth. The dog's mouth should be gently held slightly open to ensure that the strokes for the maxillary premolar and molar teeth do not also provide additional brush strokes to the mandibular premolar and molar teeth. To make the brushing process as comfortable as possible for the dog and as simple as possible for the person brushing the teeth, and depending on the size of the teeth and the size of the head of the brush, the number of teeth included in each horizontal stroke can be varied, provided that each tooth receives three back-and-forth horizontal strokes and a final vertical stroke.

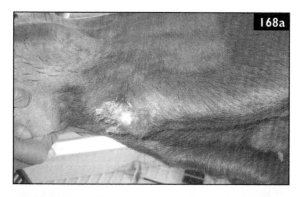

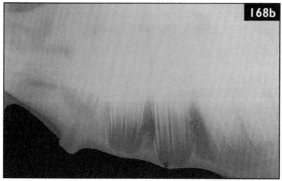

Question 168 This figure (**168a**) and radiograph (**168b**) show a 5-year-old quarter horse with a mandibular draining tract.
1 What is the diagnosis and treatment plan for this horse?
2 What long-term complication(s) should be anticipated?

Question 169 This 10-year-old, spayed female Collie (**169**) has a serum urea nitrogen of 99 mg/dl (70.3 mmol/l) and creatinine of 10 mg/dl (885 mmol/l).
1 What is the diagnosis?
2 What factors are responsible for the oral changes in this patient?
3 What treatment would benefit this patient?

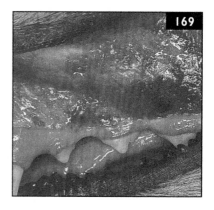

Answer 168

1 The draining tract is communicating with a non-vital left mandibular third premolar tooth. The tooth demonstrates endodontic findings of failure to narrow the pulp horns, periapical lucency, and external inflammatory root resorption. Treatment is limited to endodontic therapy or extraction. Endodontic therapy in a developing tooth, combined with a draining tract and significant apical change, has a low success rate. Further conservative management will not yield resolution as the non-vital tooth will continue to be a source of infection. The treatment of choice is oral extraction of the tooth. The extraction can be accomplished in a standing position with an inferior alveolar nerve block to desensitize the mandibular dental quadrant. A sulcular incision is made around the tooth and then luxation would be performed to cut the periodontal attachments. Careful axial movements would be performed with a molar forceps and delivery of the tooth made with the aid of a fulcrum. The draining tract would be débrided with lavage of the vacated alveolus. A postoperative radiograph should be obtained demonstrating a vacated alveolus. The vacated alveolus is packed with a suitable packing material and serial rechecks made to insure a proper healing process.

2 In the months and years following dental extractions the teeth on either side will undergo mesial drift and close the vacated space. The occluding tooth in the opposite jaw will continue to erupt without attritional wear and result in an overlong crown and malocclusion. These are major long-term implications for the oral conformation of the patient and regular occlusal adjustments, i.e. at 3–6-month intervals, is indicated to prevent secondary complications.

Answer 169

1 Uremic stomatitis. The uremic patient also has signs of systemic disease. Clinical signs associated with uremia may include depression, lethargy, halitosis ('uremic breath'), loss of appetite, weight loss, vomiting, diarrhea, and oral ulceration. Diagnostic evaluation of the uremic patient will indicate significant elevation of the serum creatinine, urea nitrogen, and phosphorus. Uremia may be secondary to postrenal disorders or renal failure (acute or chronic) with chronic renal failure the most common cause of 'uremic stomatitis'.

2 Irritation of soft tissues from ammonia produced by degradation of urea by urease-producing oral bacteria; uremic vasculitis and thrombosis resulting in necrosis and sloughing of the rostral tongue; alterations of the immune response secondary to uremia.

3 Treatment of the primary renal or postrenal problem causing the uremia should be the major focus. Decreasing the blood urea nitrogen level will decrease the urea in saliva and gingival crevicular fluid available for ammonia production. Oral pain is a significant problem in some patients and the topical application of lidocaine gel or a sucralfate paste may help to alleviate the oral pain.

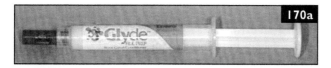

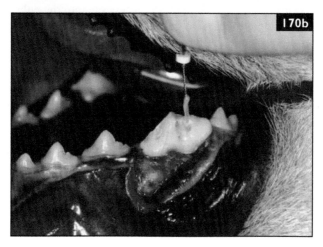

Question 170 Glyde™ File Prep Root Canal Conditioner (Dentsply Maillefer, Tulsa, OK) is a viscous liquid compound consisting of 15% ethylenediaminetetra-acetic acid (EDTA) and 10% carbamide peroxide in a water-soluble base (**170a, b**).
1 How is Glyde™ supplied, and what is its purpose?
2 How is this product used?
3 When is the liquid form of EDTA indicated?

Question 171 A 13-year-old, male castrated domestic longhair cat was presented for professional dental cleaning. The clients report that the cat is healthy and the dental disease does not appear to bother the cat; he has an excellent appetite. The cat has periodontal disease, is thin and tachycardic (>200 beats per minute), and a grade II/VI systolic murmur is auscultated over the left apex. In reviewing the medical records, the cat weighed 5.9 kg 3 years ago and presently weighs 4.5 kg.
1 What would you specifically evaluate on your physical examination?
2 What diagnostic tests are indicated?

Answer 170

1 In 3 ml curved-tip syringes. It is a chelating and lubricating material that will soften inorganic debris and lubricate the endodontic file. It is used during the initial root canal preparation.

2 Glyde™ is either deposited through the access site into the pulp chamber with the curved-tip syringe or delivered to the root canal on the tip of an endodontic file during root canal preparation in standard root canal therapy. If a bulk jar is used, a small amount is first transferred from the bulk jar to a clean sponge or a gauze pad. It is then deposited onto the file tip. Glyde™ is used either by itself or it may be used alternating, during root canal preparation, with irrigation solutions such as 2.6–5.25% sodium hypochlorite, physiologic saline solution, or other medicated solutions.

3 Liquid EDTA is used as a prefinal rinse of the canal to remove the smear layer. It is also often used throughout filing when rotary file instruments are used in place of hand files.

Answer 171

1 Palpation for the presence of a thyroid nodule.

2 The patient should have a minimum database (CBC, biochemical profile, urinalysis) and cardiac ultrasound (**171**) before general anesthesia. The signalment and history are compatible with hyperthyroidism; a serum T4 should be measured regardless of whether a thyroid nodule is present or not. More specific thyroid hormone tests or several tests obtained over time, to account for fluctuations in thyroid hormone, may be necessary to confirm the diagnosis. General anesthesia

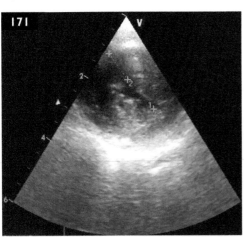

for an elective procedure should be delayed until the cat is treated for the hyperthyroidism, if present. It is also important to assess the blood pressure and evaluate the kidneys and heart in cats with hyperthyroidism. Concurrent renal disease, hypertrophic cardiomyopathy (**171**), and hypertension may need to be managed prior to anesthesia. If the cat is not hyperthyroid, an alternative explanation for the weight loss, tachycardia, and cardiac murmur should be identified.

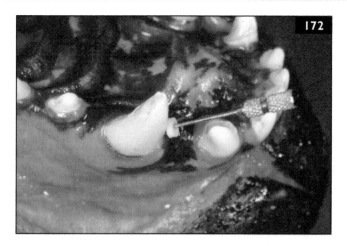

Question 172 The file is in the access site for performing standard root canal therapy on this ten-year-old Golden retriever (**172**).

1 Is the access site in the correct place?
2 What is the purpose of the yellow material pierced by the file?
3 Should the pulp chamber coronal to the access site shown be prepared and obturated in a non-fractured crown?

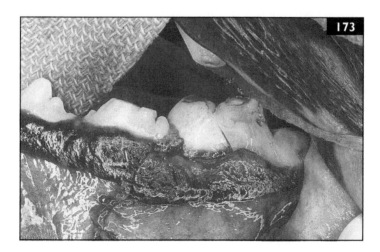

Question 173
1 Identify the periodontal surgical technique demonstrated here (**173**).
2 What are the indications for periodontal flap surgery?

Answer 172

1 Yes, although the access ideally would be made more mesially; the clinician should take into account the fact that the third incisor tooth might interfere with the head of the handpiece, obstructing clear and easy penetration of the pulp chamber. In the dog, the canine teeth are curved, so straight-line access to the apex is best made at the mesiobuccal aspect of the tooth, about 1–2 mm coronal to the gingival margin. The third incisor tooth will interfere with the access if the entrance is made too far mesially. If the entrance site is too coronal, one may place excessive stress on the endodontic file, subjecting it to unnecessary fatigue. Also there will be a tendency to over-prepare (strip) the distal aspect of the canal or gouge and perforate the mesial aspect of the canal.

2 An endodontic stop. This rubber-like material is perforated by the endodontic file before being inserted into the access hole. It is used first as a measuring device in determining the working length of the file during standard root canal preparation, and subsequently serves to assure that over-instrumentation does not occur with successive, sequentially larger files.

3 It is controversial whether the pulp chamber coronal to the main access site should be instrumented. Human endodontic texts recommend removal of all pulp chamber contents. It is generally accepted that percolation of fluids can occur from the pulp chamber. Residual bacteria, bacterial breakdown products, toxins or organic debris in the pulp chamber can therefore act as periapical tissue irritants. Many veterinary dentists believe that infection within the pulp chamber will be contained and prevented from further periapical contamination by the combined installation of root canal sealer, gutta-percha, and the intermediate restorative.

Answer 173

1 This is a periodontal flap, specifically an apically repositioned flap used for an uncomplicated crown–root fracture on the buccal aspect of the left mandibular first molar tooth. The apical repositioning is evident at the mucogingival junction. The ability to apically reposition the flap is limited by the presence of the furcation in multirooted teeth.

2 The primary indication is the presence of advanced periodontitis with deep infrabony pockets which are not fully accessible by a closed approach. Periodontal flap surgery improves the access to deep pockets and allows better visualization and therefore a greater cleanliness of the root surfaces. Secondarily, flap surgery is used as an approach for bone grafting and guided-tissue regeneration. Flaps are also indicated for the elimination of pockets through recontouring or removal of soft or hard tissue – often called 'resective therapy'. Flap surgery can also be used to reposition attached gingiva to correct the gingival contour, as in the case illustrated (**173**).

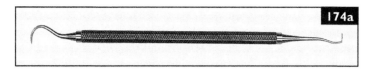

Question 174 Identify this instrument (**174a**), and compare its design with that of periodontal curettes.

Question 175

1 What are the various techniques for obtaining vinyl polysiloxane impressions (**175a**)?

2 What is the purpose of the two-step technique?

3 Briefly describe how the two-step technique is performed.

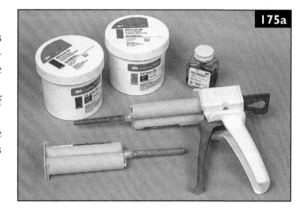

Question 176

1 What are the main problems that may be encountered with alginate impressions and that result in an unusable study model like the one shown (**176a**)?

2 How can these problems be avoided?

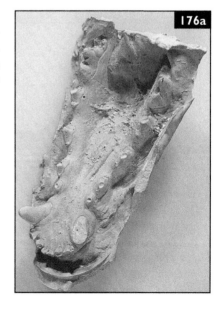

Answer 174 A Towner–Jacquette scaler, which is a double-ended instrument combining a curved and a straight sickle scaler. There are two basic types of sickle scalers: the *straight* sickle scaler (**174b**, A) and the *curved* sickle scaler (**174b**, B). The straight sickle scaler has two cutting edges on a straight blade that ends in a sharp point; this instrument is also known as a Jacquette scaler. The curved sickle scaler has two cutting edges on a curved blade. The back of a straight sickle scaler is slightly flattened, in contrast to a curved sickle scaler, which has a pointed back. Sickle scalers are designed for the removal of supragingival calculus. These instruments are used with a blade angulation of 45–90° and with a pull stroke. They are primarily used for the removal of gross supragingival calculus, e.g. before using the ultrasonic scaler, and for removal of calculus from developmental fissures, e.g. the maxillary fourth premolar tooth in the dog.

Periodontal curettes have a rounded toe and back. They can be used for supragingival calculus removal near the gingival margin, but are primarily used for subgingival scaling, root planing, and curettage of diseased pocket epithelium. There are two basic types: the *universal curette* (**174b**, C) and the *Gracey curette* (**174b**, D). The face of the universal curette is perpendicular to the terminal shank and has two cutting edges. Universal curettes can be used on both mesial and distal tooth surfaces. The face of the blade of Gracey curettes has an angulation of 70° and has only one active cutting edge. Gracey curettes are area-specific, i.e. they are designed for specific teeth and surfaces. A wide variety of universal and Gracey curettes are available, with variations in the shape and length of the shank and blade.

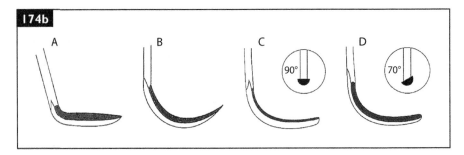

Answer 175
1 (1) The one-step putty/wash technique. (2) The two-step putty/wash technique. (3) The double-mix technique. (4) The single-mix technique.
2 The two-step over-impression will change a stock tray into a custom tray in the putty/wash technique. This reduces the large dimensional change which occurs when injection materials are used in a full-arch tray.

3 (1) An over-impression is taken with putty-type impression material and a suitable impression tray. The use of a solid tray and tray adhesive is recommended. Place only enough putty in the tray to cover the teeth (175b). Excessive putty puts pressure on the tray's side walls and increases the chance of distortion. (2) Wiggle the tray in the mouth before the putty has set to create an enlarged over-impression. After the putty has set, remove the tray from the mouth. (3) After a clean, dry field is achieved, apply a small amount of light-body impression material or 'wash' around the tooth that is being prepared for a crown restoration as well as a thin coat (1–2 mm thick) over all the teeth to be included in the over-impression. An air syringe can be used to blow the impression gently into the sulcus. Note that the wash material should not be placed over the palate. Impression material in the palate will shrink because of the bulk and distort the lingual margins of prepared teeth. (4) To seat the impression, apply very light pressure and allow the filled impression tray to slowly settle into place. Slightly pull on the lips so that the excess material can gently flow out from underneath the tray passively with no compression until completely set. If an elastomeric impression is removed before it is completely set, it will distort. (5) Remove the

impression in a rapid movement down the long axis of the teeth. (6) Inspect the impression: the margin of the prepared tooth must be entire and the crown preparation distinct and without defects. If any putty shows through in the preparation area, the impression should be taken again. Exposed set putty creates a pressure spot which will rebound when the impression is removed and result in a casting that is too small.

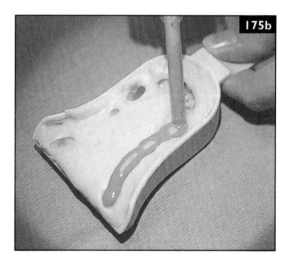

Answer 176

1 Too grainy material; tearing; air bubbles; irregularly shaped voids; distortion.
2 *Grainy alginate* can be avoided by proper mixing technique; the amount of alginate needed for the size of the tray should be measured. Cold water will slow down the set of the alginate and therefore increase the working time; conversely, warm water will speed up the set and decrease the working time. All the water

should be added to the alginate at one time. Pour the water into the premeasured powder, stirring slowly with the spatula (**176b**). Once the powder is wet, vigorously swirl the wet alginate against the sides of the bowl until there are no lumps of powder left in the mixture. This process should be completed in less than 1 minute. *Tearing* can be caused by inadequate bulk, moisture contamination, premature removal, and prolonged mixing. To avoid inadequate bulk, a tray of the correct size should be used. The tray should fit the animal's mouth, allowing room for all the teeth, without making contact with the impression tray. *Air bubbles* can be avoided by using the correct technique, avoiding the incorporation of bubbles during spatulation and loading the tray. *Irregularly shaped voids* can be prevented by ensuring that the impression is clean and free of debris. Therefore, saliva and dental calculus should be removed. A final rinse and dry should be done immediately before the impression is taken. *Distortion* can be prevented by holding the tray steady in the mouth until the alginate has set; this is very important. The alginate will set in approximately 3–7 minutes, depending on the type used. Touching the alginate around the top of the impression tray periodically can help to determine when it has set. To remove the

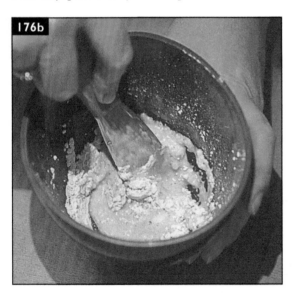

tray, grip the front of the tray and firmly snap it off. Premature and improper removal will cause distortion. Once the desired impression is obtained, the stone can be poured immediately. If pouring is delayed, the impression should be wrapped in a dampened paper towel and refrigerated. Alginate is sensitive to air, heat, and loss of moisture, so the stone should be poured within 30 minutes and the cast should be left to set for 2 hours.

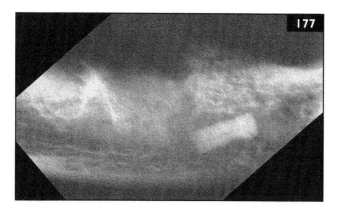

Question 177 Dental extractions do not always go according to plan. What course of action would be most appropriate in the following circumstances?
1 Following full periodontal therapy, attempted extraction of an otherwise healthy tooth root has forced it into the mandibular canal in an 18-year-old cat (**177**).
2 Continuing minor hemorrhage from the alveoli 5 minutes after closed extraction of periodontally diseased incisor teeth in a dog.

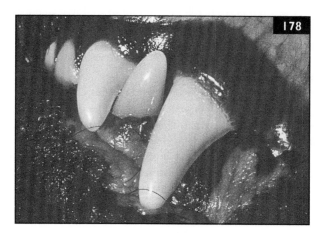

Question 178
1 What is the most likely cause of the discoloration of the teeth in this 2-year-old dog (**178**)?
2 Describe the development of this condition.
3 How can the color vary in this condition?
4 How can this condition be prevented?

Answer 177

1 It is generally stated that all root remnants should be removed; however, the whole patient must be considered. Extraction of the root in this case would considerably prolong anesthesia, with associated risks to the patient. The root was healthy and the attempted extraction was being performed in a cleaned mouth. In such circumstances it would be reasonable to leave the root where it was, close the gingiva over the alveolus, obtain a radiograph for future comparison, advise the owners of the problem, and arrange follow-up. With an infected root tip there is a serious risk of abscessation or osteomyelitis so it would be more appropriate to obtain surgical access through the bone directly over the displaced tooth root for its removal.

2 In most cases, hemorrhage from incisor tooth extraction alveoli will not be a serious problem. Application of direct pressure with a damp swab and/or cold compresses and/or suture placement to close the gingiva across the affected alveoli are likely to control the hemorrhage. Additionally, the use of tissue-compatible hemostatic agents, such as oxidized regenerated cellulose, placed loosely into an affected alveolus, can be beneficial. It is a good idea to perform a bleeding test before surgical procedures which have the potential for hemorrhage. A simple method of screening for problems involves stabbing the mucosal surface of the lip or cheek with a hypodermic needle or a special 'mucosal bleeding test' device. In animals with adequate hemostasis, bleeding will stop within 2.6 minutes, often much less. This is not entirely reliable and more sophisticated tests should be performed in breeds with recognized clotting defects.

Answer 178

1 Tetracycline staining.

2 Tetracycline reacts with calcium to form a tetracycline–calcium orthophosphate complex. In the period of mineralization during the development of teeth, tetracycline administration can cause permanent discoloration of the hard dental tissue in the deciduous and permanent dentitions. The location of the pigmentation in the crown coincides with the part of the tooth developing at the time of administration of tetracycline. The longer the administration the wider the area affected: the discoloration may vary from diffuse bands of varying widths at different levels, to totally discolored crowns. Enamel defects have been mentioned in human literature.

3 The color may vary from lemon yellow (tetracycline, demeclocycline) to yellow–gray and/or brownish (chlor- and oxytetracycline). Minocycline causes a blue–grayish pigmentation. Oxytetracycline gives the least discoloration and doxycycline appears to cause very little dental discoloration. The color can change to a darker shade after exposure to light.

4 Tetracyclines can cross the placenta and are excreted with the mother's milk. To prevent discoloration of the dental hard tissues the administration of tetracyclines should be avoided during pregnancy and the development of the deciduous and permanent dentitions.

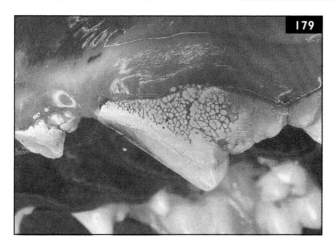

Question 179 Calculus (179) is mineralized plaque.
1 How does it form?
2 What is its composition?
3 Is calculus pathogenic?

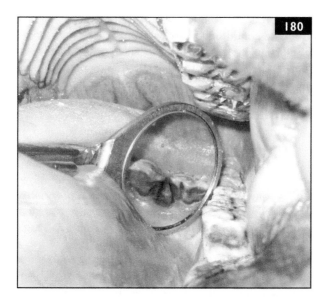

Question 180 This horse has an abnormal space between the left mandibular fourth premolar and first molar teeth (180). What is this space called and what type is it classified as?

Answer 179

1 Dental plaque serves as an organic matrix for subsequent mineralization. Precipitation of mineral salts usually begins within 2 weeks after plaque formation. The mineral source for calculus is saliva for supragingival plaque and gingival fluid for subgingival plaque. Crystals form initially in the intercellular matrix and on bacterial surfaces, and, for some specific species, within the bacteria. Calculus is formed in layers, often separated by a thin cuticle that becomes embedded in it as calcification progresses. Food debris and hair are often found incorporated in calculus in dogs. The structure is heterogeneous with a variable thickness and density. The surface is irregular and rough.

2 In humans, supragingival calculus consists of 70–90% inorganic material, mainly calcium phosphate; other salts are calcium carbonate and magnesium phosphate. The crystals formed vary according to the age and location of calculus, brushite being more common in supragingival calculus and magnesium whitlockite in subgingival calculus. The organic component consists of protein-polysaccharide complexes, desquamated epithelial cells, leukocytes, and various types of bacteria. Subgingival calculus has less brushite and more whitlockite as well as a higher ratio of calcium to phosphate. There are few studies on calculus composition in the dog and the results vary: one author found predominantly calcium phosphate, as in humans, whereas another study found calcium carbonate to be the principal mineral component. Feline dental calculus has been found to consist of carbonate-containing hydroxyapatite.

3 Calculus itself is not considered a pathogenic agent. Roughness *per se* does not cause gingivitis, and calculus without bacteria may permit an epithelial attachment to form. However, calculus does act as a retentive area of plaque.

Answer 180 A diastema is an abnormal space between teeth. Here a secondary valve diastema is present. Diastemata have been classified into primary, secondary, and senile. Primary diastemata are interproximal spaces created by an inappropriate angulation of the cheek teeth in a mesial and distal direction. The lack of angulation allows the teeth to erupt in such a way as to allow spaces to form between teeth. Secondary diastemata are due to inappropriate shape of teeth, missing teeth or supernumerary teeth, displaced teeth, and malocclusions. Senile diastemata are formed in older horses from the normal tapering of teeth toward the apex and the loss of angulation of the second premolar teeth and third molar teeth. The shape of the diastemata has been described as open or closed, with valve diastemata has a 40% reduction in width at the occlusal surface compared to the width at the gingival margin. Diastemata are considered a form of periodontal disease in the horse; further diagnostics to identify bony pocket formation, and staging of the periodontal disease with aid of radiography, are necessary.

Question 181 The gingival sulcus is a very important area (181a).

1 What are the gingival sulcus, junctional epithelium, and sulcular epithelium?

2 How does the gingival sulcus differ from a periodontal pocket?

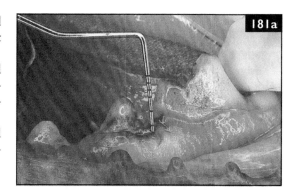

Question 182 What are the treatment options for the malocclusion in this 1-year-old dog (182)?

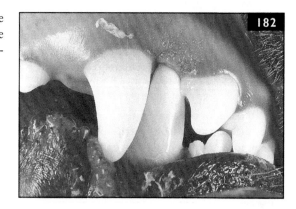

Question 183

1 Explain why this dog's malocclusion (183a) should be corrected.

2 How would you correct this malocclusion?

3 If this condition were to occur in a show prospect, how would you resolve the conflict between orthodontic treatment, American Kennel Club (AKC) regulations, and American Veterinary Medical Association (AVMA) ethics?

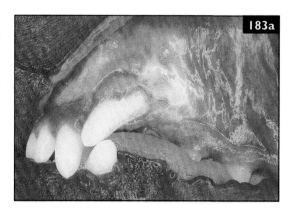

Answer 181

1 In dogs not exposed to dental plaque (germ-free dogs or dogs subjected to thorough dental home care since tooth eruption) there is no gingival sulcus (**181b, A**). The gingival margin ends on the tooth surface in a thin, narrow-angled margin with the junctional epithelium (JE) extending directly to the level of the gingival margin. This characterizes a histologically normal gingiva (no inflammation).

With plaque accumulation after tooth eruption, a sulcus forms (**181b, B**). This is the normal feature in what is called clinically healthy gingiva (not histologically healthy as a subclinical inflammation already exists). The gingival sulcus (GS) is defined as a narrow groove between the gingival margin and the tooth surface. Its depth is usually 1–3 mm in the dog and around 1 mm in the cat. The sulcular epithelium (SE) forms the lateral wall; its interior wall is formed by enamel or, with aging, by root cementum, and the bottom of the sulcus is formed by JE. The JE is located at the level of the cementoenamel junction in young dogs, whereas it is apical to it in old dogs. The interface between JE and subepithelial connective tissue follows a fairly smooth line with usually no rete pegs, contrary to the epithelial–connective tissue interface of the oral gingival epithelium. Both JE and SE are non-keratinized, although some parakeratinization is occasionally observed in SE.

2 A pseudopocket forms with gingival enlargement (**181b, C**). This should be differentiated from a true periodontal pocket (**181b, D**), which is a space around a tooth as a result of the tissue destruction which occurs with periodontitis. Both can be measured clinically by inserting a probe into the space and measuring the distance from the base of the sulcus or pocket to the free

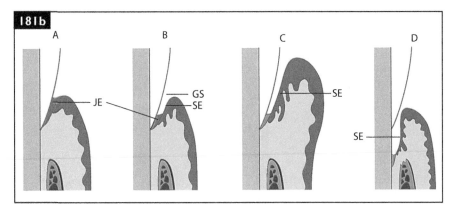

gingival margin (probing depth). A more accurate measure of attachment loss is to measure the distance from the base of the pocket to the cementoenamel junction.

Answer 182 The treatment options for linguoversion of the mandibular canine teeth and other malocclusion syndromes causing palatal trauma (see **16, 31** and **186**) include: (1) orthodontic treatment; (2) crown-height reduction; (3) alternative methods, and (4) extraction. Alternative methods include removable plastic aligners, surgical repositioning, crown extensions, and gingivoplasty combined with osteoplasty. For very minor cases ball therapy may suffice. The therapeutic decision-making is based on the severity of the malocclusion, predictability of results, required follow-up examination, desire to maintain normal structure, and expense.

Various methods for orthodontic correction of linguoversion of mandibular canine teeth have been described and are being used. An acrylic or composite inclined-plane bite plate is one of the more commonly used techniques. The appliance, which can be made by a dental laboratory based on impressions and stone models, or directly made in the oral cavity, is placed on the maxilla, which allows the palate to heal. Metal inclined planes and various types of expansion devices are also used. For minor cases, encouraging the dog to play with a suitably sized rubber ball can be successful. The disadvantages of orthodontic correction include the expense, multiple anesthesias, and plaque accumulation underneath the appliance. However, the main advantage is that the canine teeth are moved atraumatically and predictably into the correct or into a non-traumatic position.

Surgical crown-height reduction of the mandibular canine teeth to a level which takes them out of palatal occlusion, followed by vital pulp therapy or standard root canal therapy, is another option. This procedure may fail if pulp necrosis occurs. This complication makes follow-up examination imperative, even though it necessitates another anesthesia and adds to the cost.

A third option is extraction of the mandibular canine teeth. The mandibular canine teeth occupy a major part of the rostral aspect of the mandibles, and extraction weakens the structure considerably. In addition, the tongue may hang out if the mandibular canine teeth are absent.

Note that all orthodontic problems must be considered hereditary except in cases of malocclusion following known injury during development. Genetic counseling is therefore generally indicated and neutering may be recommended.

Answer 183

1 A rostrally deviated maxillary canine tooth (or so-called 'lance canine' tooth) can impair prehension and can impinge upon opposing teeth and/or the labial mucosa, resulting in occlusal and/or soft-tissue trauma. The deviated canine tooth disrupts the normal periodontal contour, thus creating a plaque-retentive area. The occlusal trauma and plaque retention increase the likelihood of focal periodontitis.

2 Orthodontic correction. Fixed dental attachments (i.e. hooks, buttons) are placed on the deviated canine tooth and on one or more anchor teeth (**183b**). The maxillary fourth premolar and the maxillary first molar teeth are often used as anchor teeth. Elastic traction (i.e. power chain, rubber bands) creates constant force on the canine tooth. The force is a mesiodistal tipping around a buccolingual axis. Commonly employed appliances consist of hooks or buttons with a power chain or rubber band stretched between them.

3 The AKC dog show rules state that altering the natural appearance of a dog for the purpose of correcting an abnormality is cause for disqualification of that animal. The AVMA states that performing a procedure for the purpose of concealing a congenital or inherited abnormality that sets the animal apart from the breed standard is unethical. Specifically, any procedure that will alter the natural dental arch is considered unethical. Should the health or welfare of the individual patient require correction of such genetic defect, it is recommended that the patient is neutered. Genetic counseling is indicated to discourage repeat breeding.

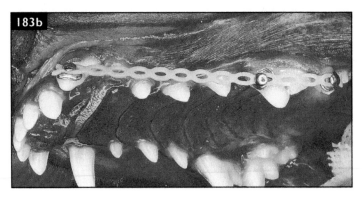

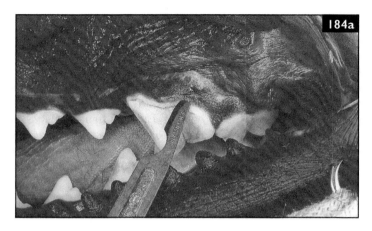

Question 184 What is the importance of the position of the gingival incision and the thickness of a periodontal flap (**184a**)?

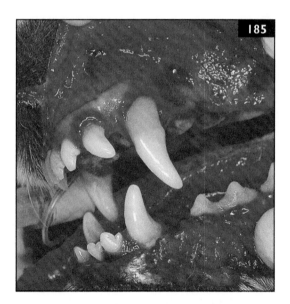

Question 185 The dog shown (**185**) has lesions limited to the oral cavity and oral mucocutaneous junctions and no systemic signs of illness.
1 Which immune-mediated diseases should be considered in this patient?
2 Which laboratory tests should be performed to diagnose immune-mediated disease in this patient?

184, 185: Answers

Answer 184 Flaps begin with a gingival incision that follows a scalloped design. The widest part of the incision is at the midpoint of the tooth, whereas the narrowest part is pointed interdentally. The further apically one wants the flap to fall, the further one makes the incision from the tooth (**184b**). Incisions which are used to elevate flaps may be intracrevicular, marginal, or submarginal depending on their proximity to the tooth. Intracrevicular incisions preserve the most soft tissue and are useful in open curettage, bone grafting, and guided-tissue regeneration surgery. With bone grafting and guided-tissue regeneration surgery, one usually attempts to preserve most of the gingiva because it is required for coverage of the site for better healing. Marginal and submarginal incisions allow the flap to fall to greater degrees of apical positioning and are useful in pocket elimination surgery. Flaps for apical positioning are made with an inverse bevel to thin the gingival margin. Pocket elimination and osseous resection for architectural revision usually

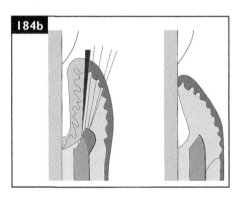

remove more gingiva by making wider and more apical incisions which end submarginally. Flaps are classified by thickness (full and partial) depending on whether epithelial covering and periosteum are included. Most surgeons prefer full-thickness flaps as split-thickness flaps interfere with the blood supply and are technically challenging. Full-thickness flaps have the advantage of better vitality because vascularity is less compromised.

Answer 185

1 Pemphigus vulgaris and bullous pemphigoid are immune-mediated skin diseases in which oral lesions are frequently found. Oral involvement, which may include gingivitis, stomatitis, and glossitis, occurs in approximately 90% of patients with pemphigus vulgaris and may be the initial manifestation of the disease in about 50% of cases. Lesions of the skin and/or mucocutaneous junctions are present with bullous pemphigoid; approximately 80% of patients develop oral lesions at the initial onset of disease or later during the course of disease.

2 Histologic and immunologic examination of oral gingival and mucosal biopsies should be obtained. Multiple biopsy specimens should be obtained from early lesions to increase the likelihood of identifying the characteristic histologic and immunologic lesions. Immunologic examination of the biopsy specimen is done to demonstrate immunoglobulin and/or complement deposition at characteristic sites for each of the immune-mediated diseases. Consultation with the diagnostic laboratory before sample collection is recommended to determine correct sample collection and handling for optimal diagnostic value.

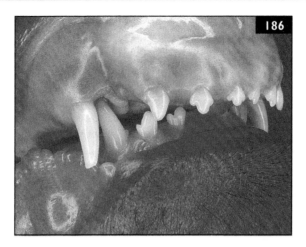

Question 186 Developmental abnormalities are commonly seen in puppies.
1 Describe the abnormality shown (**186**).
2 What is the most common cause of this type of abnormality?
3 Why is immediate treatment required, and what are the aims of treatment in a puppy?
4 What is the most practical treatment in this puppy?

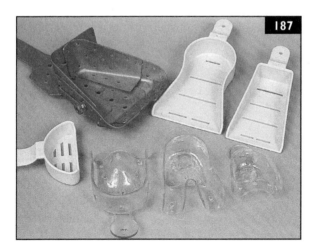

Question 187
1 Why is an impression tray used (**187**)?
2 What are the important characteristics of impression trays?

186, 187: Answers

Answer 186
1 The puppy has a pronounced mandibular brachygnathism or class 2 distocclusion resulting in malocclusion of the deciduous dentition. The mandibular incisor teeth occlude against the incisive papilla and the mandibular canine teeth are damaging the palate on the mesiopalatal aspect of the maxillary canine teeth.
2 Jaw length is determined primarily by heredity. The actual length attained by the jaw is also influenced by factors such as diet, metabolic disease, traumatic injury, infection, and both natural and artificial orthodontic forces. These factors rarely cause dramatic, symmetric changes in the mandible alone.
3 Palatal and incisive papilla contact by the mandibular canine and incisor teeth leads to discomfort, ulceration, and pain. The abnormal dental interlock with the tips of the mandibular canine teeth embedded in the palate will also interfere with further growth of the mandibles. The maxilla and mandible grow at different rates and may have growth spurts at differing times. Development of an abnormal dental interlock, whether simply due to eruption of teeth during a growth spurt or due to a jaw deformity, results in abnormal forces affecting the upper and lower jaws, restricting or enhancing growth depending on the direction of the forces. Early relief of an abnormal dental interlock may permit the jaws to grow to their full genetic potential. It must be remembered that the genetic potential may be for further deterioration of, rather than an improvement in, the situation.
4 Interceptive orthodontic extraction is the most practical treatment. It gives rapid relief from palatal trauma and removes the abnormal dental interlock. All the teeth which have an abnormal interlock or are causing palatal injury/irritation should be extracted, preferably by 12 weeks of age. Great care is required during extraction in order to minimize the risk of damaging the developing permanent tooth buds. A surgical approach is often preferable to closed extraction. It is generally recommended that extractions are performed in a bilaterally symmetric pattern so that both sides of the jaw are equally influenced by the resultant changes in functional forces.

Answer 187
1 An impression tray is used to prevent distortion while taking the impression and when pouring the stone model.
2 The most important characteristic of an impression tray is that the tray must be tri-dimensionally stable. If the tray is not rigid enough, the hydraulic pressure will displace the tray; when the impression is removed, the memory of the tray will rebound to its original dimension, making the impression smaller than the actual teeth. A proper fit should be ensured. The tray should have sufficient depth to allow impressions of the full length of the canine teeth, and large enough to perform full-mouth impressions without the tray contacting the teeth. A perforated tray is used for alginate while a solid tray combined with tray adhesive is used for other impression materials.

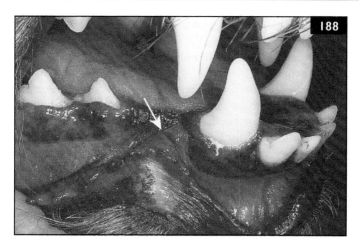

Question 188

1 Identify this structure (**188**, arrow).

2 Where in the oral cavity are there other similar structures?

3 What surgical procedure(s) is (are) occasionally performed on this structure, and why?

Question 189 This nine-year-old dog was referred for treatment of suspected chronic stomatitis and an oronasal fistula (**189**). Multiple courses of antibiotic treatment, oral rinses, and corticosteroids had not been successful in resolving the problem. What course of action is indicated?

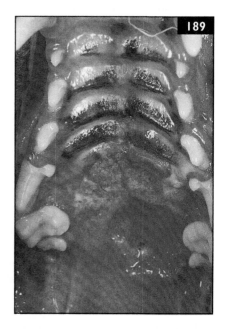

Answer 188

1 The buccal lower lip frenulum.

2 The paired buccal upper lip frenula, the single midline upper and lower lip frenula, and the tongue frenulum.

3 The procedures performed to correct impingement of the frenulum on the gingival margin are frenectomy and frenotomy. Abnormally high insertion relative to the gingival margin may be of developmental origin. Alternatively, recession of the gingival margin from disease can cause frenulum impingement and result in further recession, especially where thin gingiva and little alveolar bone overlies a prominent root. Although 'muscle impingement' has been implicated, most frenulum attachments merely transmit tension from more apically located facial muscles.

Frenectomy means removal of the frenulum from the raised surface all the way to the bone. An incision is made from mucosal surface to bone along the entire length of the frenulum and the intervening muscle, connective, and elastic tissue is excised. Frenotomy means incision through the frenulum, usually adjacent and parallel to the attached gingiva. The incision may be partial thickness or full thickness. It usually cuts across the frenulum whereas the frenectomy incision usually parallels the frenulum. Because the fibers are removed in frenectomy, the wound may be closed from side to side with sutures.

Frenotomy incisions are often not closed so that the fibers do not rejoin and recreate tension on the gingival margin. Alternatively, the sagittal frenotomy incision may be sutured in a transverse fashion. Compared with frenotomy, frenectomy appears to be more predictable in correcting the problem.

Answer 189 A complete physical examination should be performed and a minimal database established. An examination under general anesthesia can then be performed. Careful probing and intraoral radiographs are indicated to determine the extent of the bony defect underlying the oronasal fistula and to establish whether any nasal pathology is present. Computed tomography is the diagnostic imaging modality of choice. The most important diagnostic procedure includes taking one or more incisional biopsies of representative areas of the ulcerated tissue. Palpation and fine-needle aspirate of the regional lymph nodes (the mandibular lymph node in particular) is also indicated. Exfoliative cytology may be useful, but probably not bacteriologic examination, though this can be performed for the sake of academic completeness.

Multiple biopsies of this case were diagnosed as squamous cell carcinoma with ulceration and deep infiltration. Given the extent and the diffuse nature of the disease, euthanasia was advised. This case illustrates the wide spectrum of clinical presentation of oral squamous cell carcinoma (see **193**). Both in the dog and cat, chronic ulcerative lesions should always be biopsied to exclude the possibility of squamous cell carcinoma. However, care should be taken in reading out biopsies of chronic stomatitis, as epithelial hyperplasia and metaplasia associated with the latter condition may be over-interpreted and confused with neoplasia.

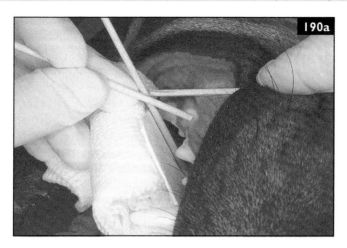

Question 190

1 What radiographic technique is being used here (**190a**) for taking a radiograph of the maxillary fourth premolar tooth in a dog?
2 Describe the geometric principle involved and positioning used in this technique.

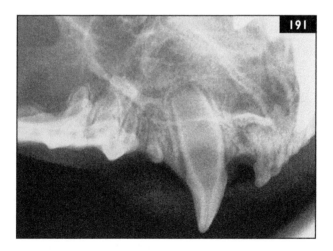

Question 191

1 Describe the radiologic findings shown (**191**).
2 Is there any pathology present in this cat? If so, describe the abnormality and suggest the cause.
3 How would you determine if the described lesion(s) is (are) associated with disease?

Answer 190

1 The bisecting angle technique is depicted (190b), which is one of the two basic intraoral radiographic techniques, the parallel technique being the other (see 41). Because of the morphology of the oral cavity, the lack of a vaulted palate in particular, the film cannot always be placed parallel to the teeth being radiographed. If the film and the teeth cannot be positioned parallel to each other, the image on the film will either be shorter or longer than the actual teeth. To obtain a radiographic image on the film which is equal in length to the teeth, the bisecting angle technique is used.

2 The bisecting angle technique involves the application of the geometric principle of equilateral triangles. In equilateral triangles, if two triangles share a side and both have an equal angle at their apex, then the opposite sides are the same lengths. When utilizing the bisecting angle technique, the intraoral film is placed in a position to allow for projection of the tooth onto the center of the film. The angle formed by the intraoral film and the long axis of the tooth is visualized. An imaginary line bisecting this angle is visualized. The central X-ray beam is then directed perpendicular to this line, which is the case when the flat end of the cone is parallel to the bisecting angle.

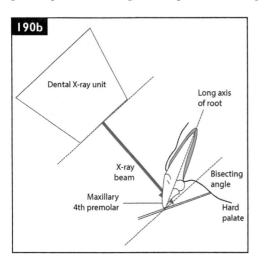

Answer 191

1 An immature tooth. The pulp chamber and root canal are wide and there is only a thin layer of dentin present. Tooth root development is incomplete. Tooth root length and apical closure have yet to be achieved.

2 In this instance there is no obvious pathology. The tooth is healthy on clinical examination and the extent of tooth root development is as expected in a young cat. The incomplete root development with an open apex is often mistaken for a pathologic lesion. If this radiograph had been of a canine tooth in an adult cat, it would have represented pathology. A vital pulp is required for continued tooth root development. Consequently, injury resulting in pulpal necrosis would have stopped tooth root development and tooth maturation and an immature tooth would have been present in the mature/adult animal.

3 If one suspects pulpal pathology, a contralateral radiograph would be indicated to determine if both teeth were at the same stage of development.

Question 192
1 What is the dental pathology demonstrated in the radiograph (**192a**) of this
older horse?
2 What treatment is indicated?

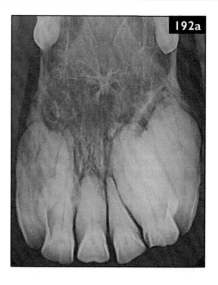

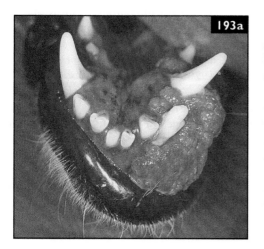

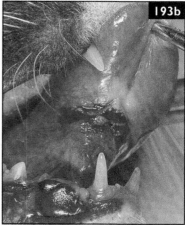

Question 193 These are two histopathologically confirmed squamous cell
carcinomas (**193a, b**). How would you summarize the clinical presentation and
biologic behavior of this tumor type in the dog and cat?

Answer 192

1 Resorption with hypercementosis of the right maxillary first, second and third incisor teeth and left maxillary second and third incisor teeth is present.

Hypercementosis is production of excess cementum surrounding the reserve crown and root of the tooth. Tooth resorption is noted along with an increased width of the periodontal ligament space. Significant bone loss has occurred at the apex of the teeth with a production of excess cementum.

2 Extraction of these teeth can be accomplished in a standing position with dental nerve blocks. The extraction process is performed as a simple extrac-

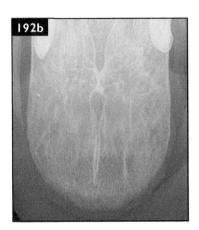

tion with a sulcular incision followed by luxation of the teeth and delivery with a forceps designed to grasp equine incisor teeth. Frequently a vertical incision of the mucosa must be performed to allow delivery of the tooth with hypercementosis due to the increased size at the apex. Closure of the incision is performed with an absorbable monofilament material in a simple-interrupted pattern. The use of bone augmenting materials is not necessary as follow-up radiographs will likely demonstrate the bone returning to a near normal anatomical level by one year (192b).

Answer 193 The gross appearance of oral squamous cell carcinoma (SCC) may vary from prominent exophytic lesions to flat, ulcerative lesions. As can also be seen in **189**, chronic oral ulceration or non-healing wounds are suspicious for SCC and should be biopsied. Bone infiltration is variable in the dog but usually very prominent in the cat, with relatively little of the tumor being visible in the oral cavity. The radiologic findings of SCC also greatly vary from minimal bone involvement to patterns dominated by bone destruction or new bone formation.

The biologic behavior of SCC is very species- and site-dependent. In general, SCC in the cat carries a much worse prognosis compared with the dog, with local recurrence due to deep infiltration being the most important cause of treatment failure. Regional lymph node and distant metastasis of SCC of the gingiva is rare, while metastasis of tonsillar and sublingual SCC is common. In general, SCC of the rostral part of the oral cavity is associated with the best prognosis, not only because of its biologic behavior but also because it is technically easier to obtain tumor-free surgical margins. The response of SCC to radiation therapy is good in the dog and poor in the cat.

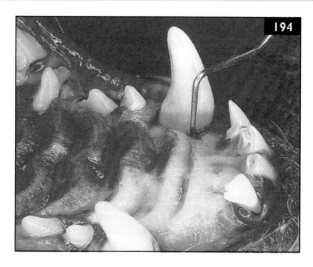

Question 194 Describe this lesion (194) and the clinical picture associated with it, and suggest methods of treatment.

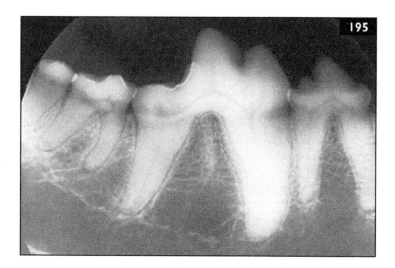

Question 195
1 What anatomic variation is evident on this radiograph (195)?
2 On which other teeth in the dog and cat is the same anomaly occasionally seen?
3 What is the clinical importance of this condition?

209

Answer 194 An infrabony pocket resulting from periodontitis on the palatal aspect of a dog's maxillary canine tooth. These pockets are typically crescent-shaped with the widest part centered on the mid-palatal surface. The lesion usually ends in a pointed fashion at the mid-mesial and mid-distal aspect of the canine tooth. Clinically, these lesions are often seen in older dolichocephalic and small-breed mesaticephalic dogs, such as dachshunds and toy poodles. There may be a unilateral purulent or serohemorrhagic nasal discharge and sneezing or coughing during eating and drinking. Typically, the gingival margin is preserved near the cementoenamel junction on the palatal surface due to the flat palatal architecture. Usually, the soft tissue of the gingival margin is only slightly inflamed and well adapted to the tooth because the most active disease process is much deeper. The lesions are usually discovered on periodontal probing rather than visual inspection and may even be difficult to detect on radiographs. The pockets are often quite deep (more than one-half the length of the canine tooth) and there may be nasal bleeding on probing when the palatal bone of the alveolus has been resorbed to the level of the nasal mucous membrane.

Treatment depends on the extent of the disease. Guided-tissue regeneration is an option for cases where an oronasal fistula is not yet present. If present, surgical extraction and soft-tissue closure is the treatment of choice.

Answer 195

1 The mandibular first molar tooth has a supernumerary root in the furcation area. Supernumerary roots generally present as a small third root in teeth that normally have only two roots. The most commonly affected tooth is the maxillary third premolar tooth (see **225**).

2 Other teeth, e.g. the mandibular fourth premolar, first molar, or second molar teeth, are rarely affected. The mandibular third molar tooth occasionally has two roots instead of one; this is more a double formation rather than a true supernumerary root. Supernumerary roots also occur in the cat, also mainly on the maxillary third premolar tooth. In one study, this condition was noted in 10.3% of maxillary third premolar teeth; the size of the extra root in these teeth varied from near normal to slender. The maxillary first molar tooth in the cat may have one or two roots.

3 A supernumerary root may be regarded as an incidental finding in the absence of other pathology. Occasionally, the supernumerary root distorts the normal gingival contour, giving rising to periodontitis. A supernumerary root is clinically important when endodontic treatment or extraction of the tooth involved is indicated. A supernumerary root, even a small one, has a root canal that forms part of the tooth's endodontic system. Failure to recognize this anomaly when endodontic treatment is indicated, and subsequently leaving this root untreated, may result in failure of the endodontic treatment. The presence of a supernumerary root complicates an extraction procedure and the tooth needs to be sectioned accordingly. This is one reason why pre-extraction radiographs are required (see also **126**).

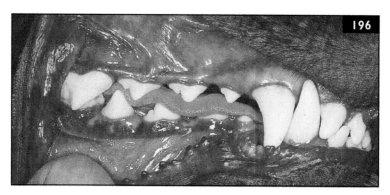

Question 196 What are the elements of a complete 'bite' evaluation in the dog (196)?

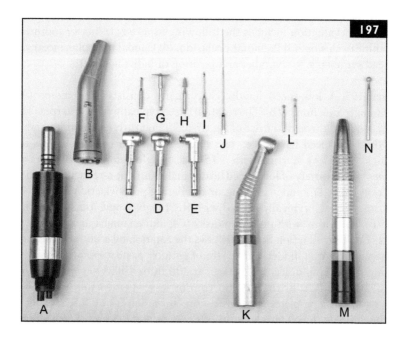

Question 197 List and describe the handpieces and types of burs pictured here from left to right (197).

196, 197: Answers

Answer 196 Normal occlusion implies normal interdigitation of teeth, integrity of the dental arches, and normal functioning of the temporomandibular joints. The normal interdigitation of teeth, or 'bite', of a dog is characterized by the anisognathous relationship of the two dental arches (the lower jaw is slightly shorter and narrower) and can be described as follows: (1) The incisal edge of the mandibular incisor teeth occludes against the cingulum of the maxillary incisor teeth (a *scissor bite*). (2) The mandibular canine tooth is centered between the maxillary canine and third incisor teeth, without touching either of them. (3) The middle cusps of the crowns of the mandibular premolar teeth fit into the interdental spaces of the maxillary premolar teeth, with each mandibular premolar tooth placed mesial to its maxillary counterpart. (4) The palatal surface of the maxillary fourth premolar tooth occludes with the buccal surface of the mesial part of the mandibular first molar tooth; the occlusal surface present on the distal part of the mandibular first molar tooth occludes with the occlusal surface of the maxillary first molar tooth.

From the above, it is clear that the evaluation of the interdigitation of teeth should not only include the incisor teeth, but the canine and premolar teeth as well. A full orthodontic evaluation includes the following aspects: (1) Incisor tooth occlusion. (2) Canine occlusion. (3) Premolar occlusion. (4) Caudal premolar/molar occlusion. (5) Head symmetry. (6) Number and position of individual teeth.

Answer 197 A low-speed handpiece typically consists of a motor (A) and a contra-angle attachment (B). The rotation speed typically is 20,000 rpm. The slower speed, acquired through the use of a gear-reduction turbine, provides higher torque than the high-speed handpiece. The contra-angle attachment changes the working angle by 75° by starting with a 15° back angle before its 90° working angle. It comes with a variety of low-speed heads, including a non-reduction head (C), a 1:4 reduction head (D), and a rotating or oscillating prophylactic head (E). The non-reduction head (C) typically is used with RA (Right Angle) burs with a latch-type shaft (F), a mandrel with polishing disks (G), and enamel and amalgam polishing points (H). The reduction head (D) slows the rotation by a set ratio, i.e. 1:4 or 1:10 for use with Gates–Glidden burs (I) and Lentulo® paste carriers (J).

A high-speed handpiece (K) rotates at 300,000–400,000 rpm when not under a load. Its speed drops to 100,000 rpm or less when cutting tooth. It has low torque and will completely stall if too much pressure is applied during use. The bur chuck holds the bur in the head of the handpiece. Some older handpieces use a chuck key, while most current ones have a push-button feature to allow quick bur changes. Some have fiberoptic or LED lights to add illumination directly to the bur's working site. FG (Friction Grip) burs (L) are available in regular, short shank, long shank, or surgical length (very long shank).

The straight or surgical handpiece (M) is a low-speed handpiece that accepts HP (Handpiece) burs (N) used for surgical procedures (e.g. osteotomy), occlusal adjustments in rabbits and rodents, and laboratory procedures.

Question 198 The crown of this dog's maxillary fourth premolar tooth (**198**) was fractured and the pulp chamber was exposed. It is not known when the injury occurred.

1 Describe the radiologic findings.
2 What is the most likely etiology?
3 What are your treatment options?
4 What follow-up treatment would you recommend?

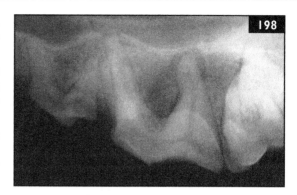

Question 199

1 'Left' and 'Right' markers are generally not used on conventional dental films, contrary to conventional radiography. If the embossed dot (not visible) on the film is facing up, which part of the dog's dentition is this (**199a**)?
2 In general, how can the teeth on dental films taken of a dog be identified?
3 Is this any different in the cat?

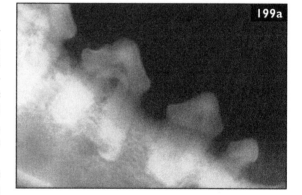

Question 200 These are three instruments used for periodontal surgery (**200a**).

1 Identify each instrument.
2 What is the intended use for each instrument?

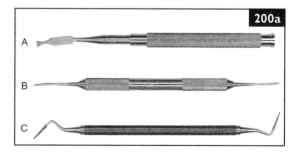

Answer 198

1 The complicated crown fracture, i.e. where the pulp is exposed in the fracture line, is evident on the radiograph. There is a distinct, rounded, radiolucent area associated with the apex of the distal root. Apical rarefaction on a radiograph usually indicates the presence of soft tissue around the tooth root apex. Such tissue can be a granuloma, cyst, or abscess. Although the radiologic signs are often suggestive of the type of lesion, definitive differentiation between these three entities relies on histopathologic examination of the tissue.

Not all apical rarefaction is pathologic in dogs and cats. The periapical bone of healthy canine teeth often appears radiolucent in the dog. Comparison should always be made with other teeth of the same type in the same animal. A distinctly round radiolucent area, however, is usually pathologic.

2 The periapical lesion seen is the result of an irreversible pulpitis or pulp necrosis resulting from the traumatic pulp exposure. Periapical lesions result as an inflammatory response to chronic pulpitis or necrotic, and generally infected, pulp. Bacteria play a key role in the pathogenesis of periapical lesions, even though bacteriologic culture often yields no growth.

3 Treatment options include extraction and endodontic therapy (see 204). If there is evidence of periodontitis in addition to the endodontic lesions, then extraction is generally the treatment of choice. Endodontic therapy should be limited to periodontally sound teeth.

4 In the case of endodontic therapy, the result of the treatment needs to be checked radiographically 3–6 months postoperatively and then annually (see 61). If the treatment has been successful, the periapical radiolucency should have filled in or be filling in with bone. If the radiolucency is getting larger, this indicates that there is still an ongoing inflammatory process resulting in bone destruction. The most likely cause of this happening is that inflamed or necrotic pulp tissue is still present in the apical segment of the root. Treatment options now include further endodontic therapy or extraction of the tooth.

Answer 199

1 The premolar region of the right mandible.
2 Dental films have an embossed dot on one corner pointing toward the X-ray source. Given the fact that the dot must have faced toward the X-ray source, there is only one way that the film could have been placed in the mouth. This enables you to orient processed dental films as to left side/right side. By orienting the embossed dot towards you ('bubble up'), you will be observing the dentition from the outside. With labial mounting, the set of whole-mouth films is spread out on the view box with the patient's midline in the center (199b). The patient's dentition will be spread out such that films to your right will be the patient's left side and films to your left will be the patient's right side,

as (generally) on a dental chart. Orienting films with the embossed dot up assumes that intraoral technique was used; this is the case for all recommended standard views in the dog. The first step when identifying a set of films is to place all films with the embossed dot up. Subsequently, mandibular films are placed on the lower half of the view box, and maxillary films on the upper half. Useful landmarks are the palatine fissures, floor of the nasal cavity, three-rooted teeth (maxilla), and mandibular canal. Next, the maxillary films are oriented such that crowns point down, and mandibular films such that crowns point up. Left from right can now be determined by identifying the molar teeth distally and the premolar teeth mesially.

3 Intraoral technique is also recommended in the cat, except for the caudal maxilla (see **221**). If the extraoral, near-parallel technique is used for the maxillary premolar and molar teeth in the cat, these films should be placed on the view box with the embossed dot down.

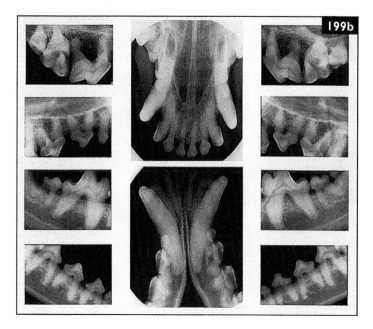

Answer 200
1 A. Ochsenbein #1 bone chisel; B. Kramer–Nevins #1/2 bone chisel; C. Sugarman 3S/4S periodontal file
2 The Ochsenbein #1 and Kramer–Nevins #1/2 are bone chisels that are used for performing the initial bulk ostectomy of the alveolar margin bone with type II crown lengthening, or with resective periodontal surgery for the removal of vertical

215

bone defects (**200 b, c**). Delicate bone chisels are preferable over power rotary instruments for this purpose to avoid damage to the root surfaces and heat-related injury to the osteocytes. The Ochsenbein chisel has two semilunar notches that are beveled on each side; the Kramer–Nevins chisel has a long mono-beveled blade.

The Sugarman periodontal file is intended for breaking up/crushing larger pieces of interproximal calculus and for contouring of the interproximal bone. This file has blades on both sides of its working end, and must be used with a short pulling stroke to prevent grooving of the root surface. In the dog, the Sugarman file is typically used to clean root surfaces and remove diseased bone when performing an apically repositioned flap at the mandibular incisors (**200d**).

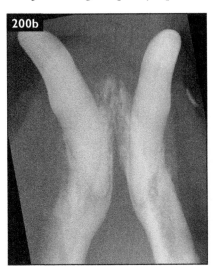

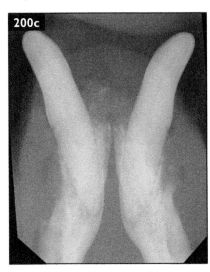

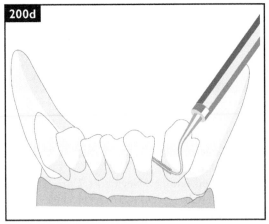

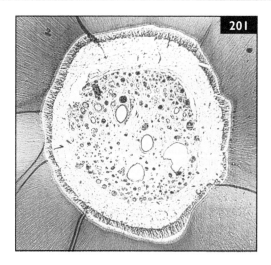

Question 201 This is a low-magnification, cross-sectional view of a dog's tooth root (201).
1 What cell layers are visible in the pulp?
2 What nerve fibers are present in the pulp, and what is their clinical significance?

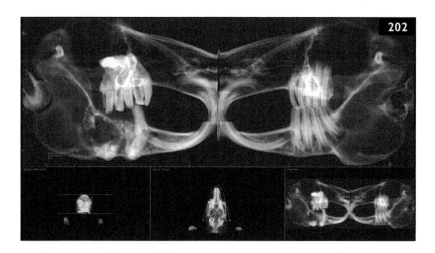

Question 202
1 What diagnostic imaging modality has been used here (202)?
2 What are the advantages of this modality?
3 What is the main disadvantage?

Answer 201

1 The most peripheral layer consists of the odontoblasts, which are closely associated with the predentin and dentin (see **97, 114** and **155**). The odontoblasts are columnar in the pulp chamber and more cuboidal in the root canal. Under the odontoblasts is the cell-free zone (of Weil), which typically is fairly wide in the dog. The next layer is the cell-rich zone, which contains fibroblasts and undifferentiated mesenchymal cells. Intertwined with this zone is the parietal nerve plexus layer (or subodontoblastic plexus of Raschkow). The fibroblasts form the pulp matrix, while the undifferentiated mesenchymal cells may become involved in the production of tertiary dentin. The pulp proper or pulp core consists of loose connective tissue and contains the large blood vessels, lymphatic vessels, and nerves.

2 The dental pulp is richly innervated and contains sensory and postganglionic sympathetic fibers, which can be divided into relatively large-diameter, myelinated A-β and A-δ fibers, and small-diameter, unmyelinated C fibers. The terminal nerve fibers lose their myelin sheath and arborize to form the plexus of Raschkow, with a few A-δ axons continuing between the odontoblasts and accompanying the odontoblastic processes in the dentinal tubules. This partially explains why dentin is sensitive. Stimulation of the A-δ fibers is responsible for momentary, sharp, provoked, and localizable pain. This is indicative of a vital pulp with an intact dentin–pulp complex. As pulpitis progresses and the pulp degenerates, C-fiber pain predominates; this is characterized by a more constant, diffuse, throbbing pain.

Answer 202

1 Cone-beam computed tomography (CBCT) has been used here to obtain a panoramic view.

2 With the help of computer software the viewer is able to scroll through the volume and simultaneously view axial, coronal and sagittal 2D sections as low as 0.15 mm in thickness, and excellent quality 3D reconstructions. This technique has been shown to be suitable for early detection of even small changes in bone and adjacent soft tissues and provides clear images of dental anatomy and pathological changes. The spatial resolution in conventional CT is usually of the order of 1 mm or just below this value. When scanning small objects, this results in images, containing a small number of pixels, resulting in a spatial resolution that is low. Compared to conventional CT, the patient ionizing radiation dose levels are kept to an absolute minimum. The scan time is a mere 18–26 seconds, allowing for decreased time under anesthesia.

3 The main disadvantage for clinical use of CBCT in animals, compared with conventional CT, is the maximum size of objects that can be scanned. For example, the NewTom 5G (NewTom, Verona, Italy) CBCT produces exceptionally high spatial resolution images with six programmable fields of view ranging from 6 × 6 cm to 18 × 16 cm. This means that animals with heads longer than 16 cm, such as large-size dogs, would not be able to be imaged with CBCT at this point.

Question 203 The use of a surgical approach can simplify and reduce the risk of complications during dental extraction. By raising a gingival or a full-thickness mucogingival flap, it becomes possible to remove some of the supporting alveolar bone in order to improve access to the tooth roots and to reduce anatomical root retention, facilitating extraction.
1 For which teeth might an 'envelope' flap prove helpful during extraction?
2 Describe a triangular mucogingival flap commonly used during extraction of a maxillary canine tooth.

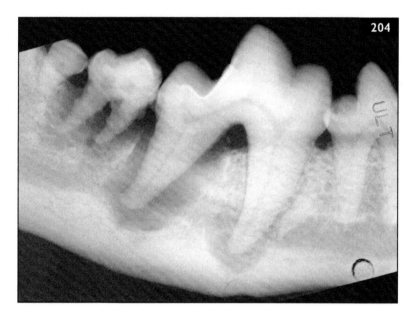

Question 204
1 Identify the pathology evident at the mandibular first molar tooth on this radiograph (204).
2 Describe how these lesions occur.
3 How are these lesions classified?

Answer 203

1 An envelope flap is made by incising through the gingival sulcus, dentogingival fibers, and interproximal gingiva of adjacent teeth, then raising the attached gingiva from the underlying alveolar bone to create a flap that does not extend beyond the mucogingival line. These flaps do not have additional releasing incisions as used in triangular and pedicle flaps. An envelope flap can be used to improve access to and visualization of the tooth root and furcation of teeth, thus assisting with instrument placement (luxators and/or elevators) during extraction and sectioning.

2 A triangle access flap is commonly used for the extraction of a maxillary canine tooth. The releasing incision in this case will start at the distobuccal line angle of the third incisor tooth, the incision being made down onto the underlying marginal alveolar bone. The incision extends around the gingival sulcus of the canine tooth, continuing interproximally to, and around, the first premolar tooth, and if necessary the second premolar tooth. A second incision is made perpendicular

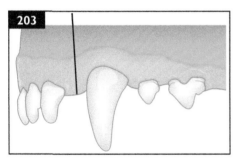

to the first, extending from the distobuccal line angle of the third incisor tooth through the gingiva and oral mucosa to just above the level of the canine tooth root apex. The gingiva and periosteum are then elevated along the length of the flap so that it can be folded back to expose the bone overlaying the canine tooth root (203).

Answer 204

1 There is a combined periodontal–endodontic lesion (*Type 2*) visible on both roots of the mandibular first molar tooth.

2 Periodontal disease and endodontic lesions can occur as combined lesions. In a periodontal disease that progresses to involve the exposure of lateral endodontic canals, open dentinal tubules on exposed root surfaces, or the apex, can result in endodontic lesions. Conversely, a periapical lesion of endodontic origin may spread periodontally. The 'true' combined lesion is when a periapical lesion of endodontic origin exists on a tooth that is also periodontally involved and the infrabony pocket extends to a point where the two lesions merge. The interrelationship of these systems can be established through the communication of the apical foramen as well as through lateral, accessory, and/or furcation canals.

3 *Type 1*: endodontic–periodontal lesions (primary endodontic lesions with secondary periodontal involvement). *Type 2*: periodontal–endodontic lesions (primary periodontal pocket(s) with secondary pulpal involvement). *Type 3*: 'true' combined lesions (concurrent primary periodontal lesions and primary pulpal lesions).

Question 205 Metal crowns should be cemented with a strong cement to achieve optimal retention.

1 Which cements have more strength and should be used for cementing metal crowns on the teeth of working dogs?

2 One step in the cementation technique of metal crowns is shown here for a three-quarter crown on a mandibular canine tooth (**205**). Describe the complete procedure.

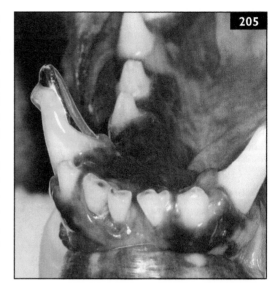

Question 206 This is an intraoperative view of a partial maxillectomy in a dog (**206**). The tumor in question was diagnosed as a squamous cell carcinoma, and mandibular lymph node palpation and thoracic radiographs showed no obvious signs of metastasis. This surgical procedure is designed to achieve a 'surgical cure'. How do you decide what to remove, and how do you go about removing sufficient tissue?

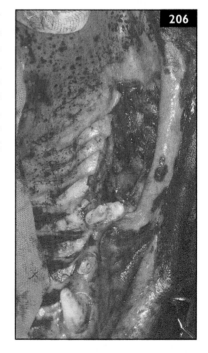

Answer 205

1 Retention of conventional prosthetic crowns is largely dependent on the preparation design (see 95). The space between the tooth surface and the metal crown should be filled with a thin layer of cement. Adhesive bonding techniques and electrolytically etching or sandblasting of the inside of the metal crown can be used to obtain the best retention. The choice of cements used to fix metal crowns on the teeth of working dogs is of importance. Composite resin cements have recently been developed and combine a high tensile and some compressive strength. They also have the capacity to bond to tooth structure. The resin Panavia-F™ cement, a composite of low viscosity, was found to be effective and provided a long-term success and adequate retention of metal crowns on canine teeth in dogs. Panavia-F cement shows good biocompatibility, no detrimental effect on the pulp, and no microleakage of the crown.

2 Before cementation the tooth should be pumice-polished, cleaned with water, and air-dried. The inside of the metal crown should be rinsed with alcohol to remove any traces of oil. After air-drying, the tooth can be etched with a 37% phosphoric acid etching gel or liquid for 30 seconds, thoroughly rinsed with water, and air-dried. The manufacturer recommends that only uncut enamel is etched. The Panavia-F cement is mixed following the manufacturer's instructions. A thin layer of the cement is applied on the internal surface of the metal crown. The metal crown is seated and the excess Panavia-F cement is removed. An oxygen inhibitor is applied to the margin of the metal crown to achieve isolation from air and thus to enable the cement to set completely (205). During the setting time the crown is kept under finger pressure for approximately 6–7 minutes.

Answer 206 The tissue must be removed 'en bloc', because there are no simple surgical limits in the maxilla to follow. For a squamous cell carcinoma, a 10 mm margin of grossly normal tissue beyond the lesion is recommended as the minimal amount to resect. Standard radiographs do not reveal sufficient detail to define three-dimensional abnormalities, especially in a complicated structure like the maxilla and nasal cavity. CT scans are more useful in this respect, though the grossly palpable and visible limits are usually the only help at hand. Once the extent of the excision is decided, incisions through soft tissue and bone are made with scalpel (for soft tissue) and osteotomy bur or osteotome (for bone) to isolate the tissue. This often requires transecting major vessels and risking extensive hemorrhage. Knowing the topographical anatomy of the major blood vessels (infraorbital artery, palatine artery, sphenopalatine artery, facial artery) is essential. If the hemorrhage cannot be stopped by pressure or identification and clamping of a specific vessel, the carotid artery on that side can be ligated. The closure of the oronasal defect created during a maxillectomy is achieved by dissecting the buccal mucosa to form a tension-free flap that is sutured to the palatal incised edge. If the buccal mucosa is not available to form a flap to cover the defect, more advanced reconstructive techniques are indicated.

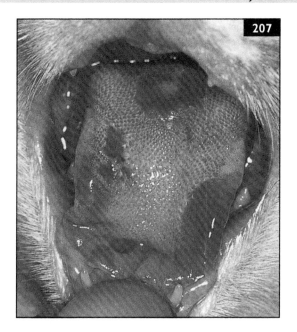

Question 207 How would you proceed with diagnosis and management of this 1-year-old cat (**207**), which is drooling and has not been eating for a few days?

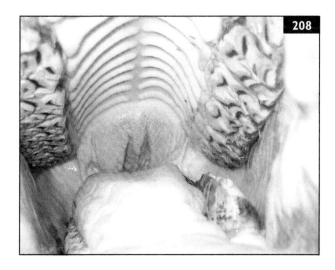

Question 208 What abnormality of the left dental quadrants is shown (**208**)?

223

Answer 207 Ulcerations of the tongue and palate are common in cats with primary acute viral infections such as herpesvirus (FHV) and calicivirus (FCV). Careful clinical examination may reveal dehydration, and other lesions (ocular and nasal discharges) that are indicative of FHV/FCV infection are usually also present. More generalized gastrointestinal signs or weakness may indicate panleukopenia viral infection. Other than viral isolation, there are no specific tests that will confirm the diagnosis of FHV or FCV infection, and there is no particular benefit to having the diagnosis confirmed (except in a cattery situation, in which issues of prevention may be very important). Lingual or palatal ulcerations resulting from FHV or FCV infection almost always heal within a few weeks of onset. The loss of condition, or in more severe cases, onset of clinical dehydration, may be obvious from results of hematocrit or CBC examinations, and panleukopenia would be an important differential diagnosis if the total white cell count is very low. To date, there is no direct evidence that FHV or FCV is a primary cause of chronic stomatitis. Calicivirus can be isolated from oral or pharyngeal fluids in many cats with chronic stomatitis (carrier status and virus replication during periods of stress for the host can account for this finding), and there are strains of calicivirus that will consistently produce caudal stomatitis lesions in specific pathogen-free cats; however, these cats do not go on to develop the chronic lesions that are so frustrating to manage. The typical cat with chronic stomatitis does not have lingual or palatal lesions. Differential diagnosis is much more important for chronic oral lesions (see **44**). Since treatment is symptomatic – nursing care, nutritional support, antimicrobial treatment to prevent secondary bacterial infections – the most important indicator is the condition and behavior of the cat. Clinically evident dehydration requires immediate management – intravenous fluid therapy if severe, or subcutaneous bolus therapy in less severe cases.

Answer 208 The occlusal table angulation is increased on the left dental quadrants of this horse. This is an acquired malocclusion that occurs when the horse avoids mastication on a particular dental quadrant. The horse has an anisognathous conformation with the maxillary quadrants anatomically wider than the mandibular quadrants. This causes a normal occlusal table angle to form which slopes downward in a lingual to buccal direction. With constant eruption of the equine cheek teeth if a particular quadrant is avoided during mastication the occlusal table angle will increase. One must identify the reason for the lack of mastication. The differential diagnosis can include a temporomandibular joint disease, fractured teeth causing soft-tissue trauma, neurologic dysfunction of the muscles of mastication, endodontic disease with pulpitis, periodontal disease with extensive food impaction, and chronic skeletal fractures of the skull. Treatment is aimed at addressing the primary cause and followed by serial occlusal adjustments aimed at correcting the occlusal table angle over several visits. Correction of the table angle in one visit may compromise the occlusal dentin thickness and cause endodontic disease of the cheek teeth.

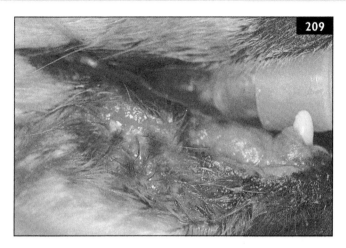

Question 209 This dog was presented for treatment of periodontal disease (**209**). The owner's primary complaint is halitosis.
1 What is the problem in this patient?
2 Which breeds are predisposed to developing this problem?
3 What dental disease may be associated with this problem?
4 What are the treatment recommendations for this problem?

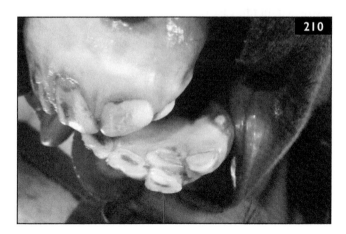

Question 210 This is a 3-year-old Quarter horse filly.
1 What dental procedure is indicated from this picture (**210**)?
2 What is the incisor tooth eruption sequence?

Answer 209

1 Lip fold dermatitis (pyoderma). Malodor from the mouth may be the result of halitosis secondary to oral disease or associated with skin or lip disease around the mouth.

2 Dogs with excessive mandibular labial tissue are commonly affected and there is a breed predisposition in the cocker spaniel, springer spaniel, St. Bernard, and Irish setter. Lip fold or skin fold dermatitis may also occur following partial mandibulectomy or maxillectomy if skin or lip folds are created during wound closure.

3 Increased plaque accumulation on teeth adjacent to the lip/skin folds may enhance the development of more severe gingivitis/periodontitis.

4 Medical treatment involves twice-daily cleaning, for 10–14 days, of the area with a benzoyl peroxide shampoo, followed by drying the area (manually or with a mild astringent), and topical application of a benzoyl peroxide gel or mupirocin ointment. Cases with severe inflammation may benefit from an initial few days of topical antibiotic/steroid cream or systemic anti-inflammatory/antibiotic administration. Unless surgically corrected, the dermatitis tends to become chronic. Benzoyl peroxide gel is applied as needed for prevention and is aimed at controlling the inflammation and preventing recurrences. Lip fold excision (cheiloplasty) should be considered in severe cases.

Answer 210

1 The left mandibular first incisor tooth is a persistent deciduous tooth and should be extracted. In this case the permanent tooth can be seen erupting behind the persistent deciduous tooth. If the permanent successor cannot be visualized a radiograph should be obtained to confirm a permanent tooth is present. If there is not a succeeding permanent tooth present and the persistent deciduous tooth is vital there is no need for extraction. A persistent deciduous incisor tooth should be extracted if any of the following conditions are present: (1) The contralateral incisor tooth is permanent and in wear. (2) The opposing incisor tooth is permanent and in wear. (3) The permanent incisor tooth has erupted behind the deciduous incisor tooth. In this case, all three conditions are present. The deciduous tooth can be extracted by elevation or luxation. The mesial aspect of the second incisor tooth should be rasped off, creating an opening so the permanent incisor tooth can move buccally, creating normal occlusion. It is also common for a fragment of an unexfoliated deciduous crown or root to remain in place. The fragment may be removed by making an incision over it, elevating the gingiva and mucosa off the fragment, and then elevating under the fragment. The wound edges are approximated with an absorbable material.

2 The incisor tooth eruption sequence is first incisor teeth: 2 years 6 months; second incisor teeth: 3 years 6 months; third incisor teeth: 4 years 6 months.

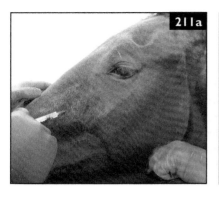
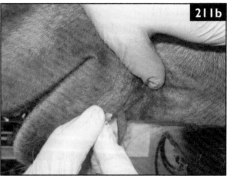

Question 211 Describe the procedures being performed in figures **211a** and **b**, and the structures that will be desensitized.

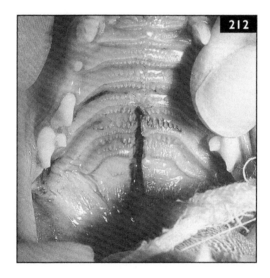

Question 212 This is an example of a traumatic condition, commonly seen in the cat (**212**).
1 What is it, and what syndrome can it be part of?
2 What are the other possible maxillofacial components of this syndrome?
3 What are the treatment options for this specific injury?

211, 212: Answers

Answer 211

In **211a** the infraorbital nerve block is being performed. The infraorbital foramen can be palpated in the horse midway between the nasoincisive notch and the medial canthus of the eye. The ventral margin of the levator nasolabialis muscles overlies the foramen and must be pushed dorsally to enter the foramen. Insertion of the needle into the infraorbital canal is necessary to cause desensitization of the nerve. The incisor, canine, premolar and, if a large enough dose is deposited, molar teeth of the maxillary dental quadrant can be desensitized. Performing this in a standing sedated horse can elicit a strong response and care must be taken to perform this block with adequate restraint. The maxillary nerve block can also be performed to desensitize the same structures. The maxillary nerve block is performed extraorally. There are several described approaches and care must be taken to avoid traumatizing the maxillary artery and causing a hematoma behind the eye.

Figure **211b** shows the middle mental nerve block. The mental nerve is a branch of the inferior alveolar nerve; the structures desensitized with the mental nerve block include the buccal mucosa, canine teeth and incisor teeth. The inferior alveolar nerve block will also block the same structures as well as the cheek teeth. The inferior alveolar nerve block in the horse has been described by two extraoral approaches and recently by an intraoral approach. When performing nerve blocks sterile technique should be followed. The inferior alveolar nerve block can have a complication of self-inflicted lingual trauma.

Answer 212

1 A traumatic cleft of the hard palate, which can be part of the so-called high-rise syndrome. This syndrome describes the injuries sustained, mainly by cats, falling at least two stories. Contrary to dogs, the survival rate in cats is high under such circumstances. A cat usually falls in a splayed-leg position and lands on all four limbs; the head then bounces against the landing surface.

2 (1) Soft-tissue facial abrasions; avulsion of the lower lip. (2) Dental fractures. (3) Mandibular fractures, in particular mandibular symphysis separation. (4) Temporomandibular joint luxation and fracture of the condylar process (see **104**).

3 Traumatic separation of the hard palate in the cat can easily and effectively be managed by approximating the displaced bony structures by gentle digital pressure, followed by suturing of the torn palatal soft tissues in a simple interrupted pattern. Flushing and suctioning the nasal cavity is indicated if large blood clots are present, which may have a marked beneficial effect on the habitus and appetite of the patient. The benefit of this initial management outweighs the risk inherent in leaving this injury to heal by second intention, although this has been shown to be sufficient in most cases. However, occasionally this healing does not take place and a persistent oronasal fistula results; the latter condition is far more difficult to manage.

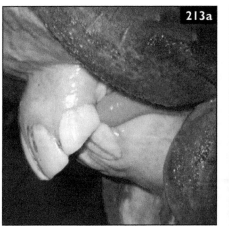
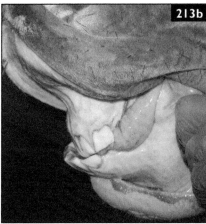

Question 213 Describe the two different malocclusions present in these figures (213a, b) and discuss areas of the dental quadrants you would expect to develop overgrowths of the dentition.

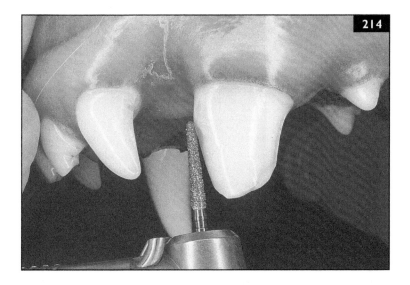

Question 214 When performing crown preparations of canine teeth (214), what anatomic features must be considered? How much tooth must be reduced?

229

Answer 213 The figures (**213a, b**) demonstrate horses with skeletal malocclusions. They each have a discrepancy in the length of the mandible in relation to the maxilla. Relative maxillary prognathia is when the mandible occludes distal to the maxilla, and may be called a class 2 malocclusion. Relative mandibular prognathia is when the mandible occludes mesially to the maxilla, called a class 3 malocclusion. In cases with relative maxillary prognathia the mesial aspect of the maxillary second premolar teeth and the distal aspect of the mandibular third molar teeth will lack opposing dentition and become overlong (**213c**). The length and width of the overlong portion of crown is proportionate to the discrepancy in jaw length. Relative mandibular prognathia would display overlong crowns

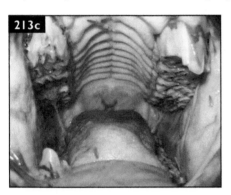

of the maxillary third molar teeth and mandibular second premolar teeth. Furthermore, the enamel folds of the teeth can cause increased wear in the interproximal spaces of the opposing quadrants promoting excessive transverse ridging in the dental quadrants of these cases. Skeletal malocclusions can also be asymmetrical with one set of opposing dental quadrants displaying the exact opposite malocclusions as noted in the picture.

Answer 214 One of the most important considerations when performing a crown preparation is the occlusion with other teeth, e.g. in the case of the mandibular canine tooth, the proximity of both the maxillary third incisor and canine tooth. The mandibular canine tooth must be reduced at the distal lingual wall to allow for clearance of the maxillary canine tooth and the mesial lingual wall for the maxillary incisor tooth. In addition, consideration should be given to allow for clearance of the soft tissues in the interdental space between the maxillary teeth. How much reduction depends on the type of crown employed. A commonly used guideline would be 0.5–1.0 mm for metal crowns and 1.5–2.0 mm for porcelain-fused metal or ceramic crowns. An additional consideration would be the shape of the tooth and the fitting of the crown afterwards. As the tooth is curved, a portion of the mesial buccal wall may have to be removed to eliminate the overhang that may exist at the gingival margin. Other considerations would be to create precise margins, and to inspect these margins and the fit before seating the crown. The crown should not have any gaps between the tooth and crown. The margin should be very smooth and free of plaque-retentive areas. If the crown has gaps greater than 0.2 mm, new impressions should be obtained and the models returned to the dental laboratory for remake.

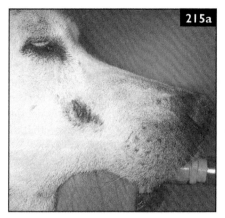

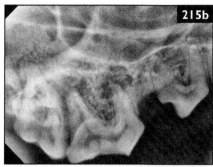

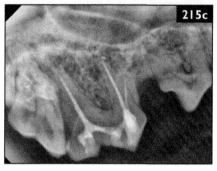

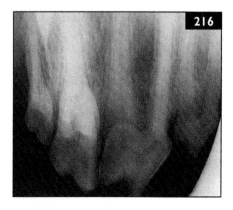

Question 215 The picture (**215a**) shows a 7-year-old dog with a right suborbital draining sinus tract. Six months ago, a root canal treatment was performed to treat a complicated crown fracture of the right maxillary fourth premolar tooth, and a similar draining sinus tract was present that resolved shortly after treatment. Radiographs at the time of initial treatment revealed well-defined peri-apical radiolucencies at all three roots, and inflammatory root resorption (**215b**).
1 What are the dental and non-dental causes for suborbital draining sinus tracts?
2 What is the most likely cause for the persistent draining sinus tract in this patient, evident on this radiograph (**215c**)?
3 What is the recommended treatment for this patient?

Question 216
1 What technical errors caused by incorrect positioning can be seen on this radiograph (**216**)?
2 Explain how the tooth length can appear incorrect on the radiograph.
3 Describe a technique for obtaining a better image of the two mesial roots of the maxillary fourth premolar tooth.

231

Answer 215

1 *Dental causes*: (1) Periapical abscessation at the right maxillary third or fourth premolar tooth, or first molar tooth. (2) Combined periodontal–endodontal lesion of any of the above three teeth. (3) If any of the above three teeth had been previously extracted, roots were fractured, and root tips were not retrieved, these retained roots could serve as a persistent source of infection. (4) Failure of root canal treatment due to residual infected periapical tissue, or an insufficiently débrided draining tract following extraction, may be recurrent sources of infection that may initially provide healing, only to return months later with similar symptoms.

Non-dental causes: (1) Soft-tissue bite wound abscess. (2) Foreign-body abscess, such as a gunshot wound or from an embedded spikelet of foxtail-type grass. (3) Maxillary fracture and bone sequestration. (4) Maxillary or nasal neoplasia. (5) Nasolacrimal duct infection or obstruction (dacryocystitis).

2 Failed root canal treatment and possible insufficient débridement of the sinus tract.

3 Follow-up dental radiographs of the root canal-treated tooth show an incomplete obturation of the palatal root, overfill with sealer puff at the palatal root, and persistent well-defined periapical radiolucencies, suggesting that healing has not occurred. Treatment options include débridement of the draining tract with surgical extraction of the tooth or surgical root canal treatment (apicoectomy with retrograde filling) of the mesiobuccal, distal roots and extraction of the palatal root.

Answer 216

1 The main error seen here is elongation. In addition, superimposition of the two mesial roots of the maxillary fourth premolar tooth is evident, which is the normal result of the standard lateral view of the maxillary fourth premolar tooth. Some cone cutting has occurred on the mesial aspect of the film, because the X-ray cone was not centered on the film or sensor.

2 Foreshortening or elongation occurs if the X-ray beam is not perpendicular to the bisecting angle plane. Foreshortening of the image may result if the X-ray beam is directed too steep, or more perpendicular to the plane of the film or sensor, similar to the shadow effect of midday sun on a tree. Elongation of the image results if the X-ray beam is directed too low, or more perpendicular to the long axis of the tooth, creating the shadow effect of early morning or late afternoon sun on a tree.

3 The standard lateral view of the maxillary fourth premolar tooth results in an image with the two mesial roots superimposed. In order to separate these two roots, an additional, slightly oblique view is indicated. 'SLOB' is an acronym for Same/Lingual – Opposite/Buccal and refers to the direction of the incoming X-ray beam as an aid in identification of roots of multirooted teeth. The root on the radiograph closest to the incoming X-ray beam is the more lingual (palatal) root. When the radiograph is obtained with the X-ray beam directed slightly from caudally, the mesiopalatal root will be projected distally to the mesiobuccal root.

Question 217 A 7-year-old, neutered male, retired racing greyhound was presented for treatment of severe periodontitis. Multiple surgical extractions were performed. Despite proper closure of the extraction sites, significant postoperative hemorrhage was observed for 24–48 hours post-surgery that required hospitalization and transfusion with both packed red blood cells and fresh frozen plasma. A hemostasis profile was obtained that evaluated both primary and secondary hemostatic pathways; this revealed a normal platelet count, as well as normal one-stage prothrombin and activated partial thromboplastin times.

1 What is the most likely cause of bleeding in this patient?
2 How can this condition be prevented?

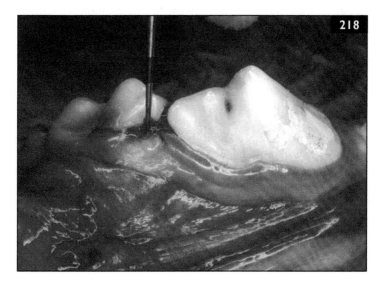

Question 218
1 What is a dental index?
2 Name and characterize one index for plaque and one index for gingival inflammation (**218**).

Answer 217

1 This complication in the greyhound, where there are no documented primary or secondary hemostatic disorders, is most likely caused by hyper- or enhanced fibrinolysis. Clot or thrombus dissolution is believed to be the cause for this complication, where excessive bleeding occurs with minor trauma or following typically routine surgical procedures such as dental extractions, neuters, and dewclaw surgeries.

2 Perioperative administration of fresh frozen plasma and/or aminocaproic acid (Amicar®) is recommended in dogs with hyperfibrinolysis. Aminocaproic acid is an anti-fibrinolytic that may decrease the severity of this complication in Greyhound dogs. The recommended dosage for aminocaproic acid is 500 mg by mouth three times daily for 5 days, and may be administered pre- and postoperatively, but also by injection intraoperatively; this medication is readily available at human pharmacies in injectable, tablet, and suspension forms for a modest cost.

Answer 218

1 An index is a numeric score based on defined diagnostic criteria. The presence and/or severity of pathologic conditions are expressed by assessing a numeric value. A wide variety of indices exist, primarily for use in humans but also for veterinary use. Some indices were developed primarily for use in epidemiologic studies, while others are more applicable to individual patients. An index should be simple, objective, reproducible, quick, and practical.

2 The Plaque Index (PI) is used to assess the thickness of plaque along the gingival margin. It uses a scale of 0 to 3. Index 0 indicates no plaque adjacent to the gingival margin. Index 1 indicates plaque adhering to the free gingival margin visible only when a probe is run across the tooth surface. Index 2 indicates a moderate accumulation of soft deposits within the gingival pocket, and on the gingival margins and/or adjacent tooth surface, which can be seen without staining or use of a probe. Index 3 indicates an abundance of soft debris at the gingival margin and interdental space.

A PI commonly used in veterinary dentistry is based on the percentage of the buccal aspect of the crown covered by plaque. An index of 1 means that up to 25% of the buccal aspect is covered by plaque, an index of 2 indicates 25–49% coverage, an index of 3 indicates 50–74% coverage, and an index of 4 indicates 75–100% coverage.

The Gingival Index (GI) is used to assess gingival inflammation. It uses a scale of 0 to 3. Index 0 indicates no inflammation. Index 1 indicates mild inflammation with slight edema, slight change in color, and no bleeding on probing. Index 2 indicates moderate inflammation with redness, edema, glazing, and bleeding on probing (218). Index 3 indicates severe inflammation, marked redness, edema, ulceration, and a tendency for spontaneous hemorrhage.

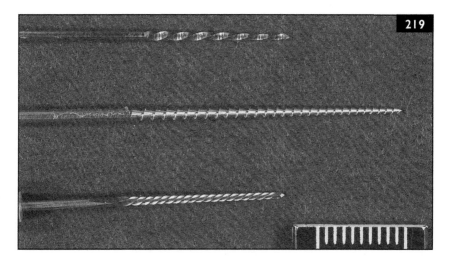

Question 219

1 Name these three types of commonly used manual endodontic instruments (**219**).
2 Describe the purpose of each, how they are fabricated and used, and their relative strength.

Question 220

1 What is the developmental abnormality (**220**) seen in this 1-year-old dog?
2 What is the clinical importance of this condition?
3 What is the identification of this tooth using the Triadan system?

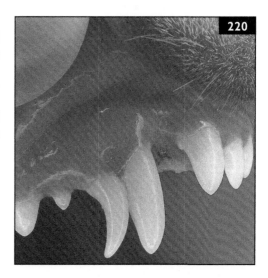

Answer 219

1 The instruments pictured are, from top to bottom, a reamer, a Hedström file, and a Kerr file or K-file.

2 Endodontic reamers and files help to remove pulp from the root canal, but they are primarily used to débride the contaminated dentin lining the root canal and to shape it for convenient filling; they are available in different styles, lengths, and diameters.

Reamers are an early edition of the file, but are still preferred by some practitioners. They are twisted, square metal rods with fewer flutes or twists per millimeter than a file. Reamers are designed to be used in a twisting, auger-like motion that carries filings from the depth of the canal to the access site.

The two most common styles of files are the Kerr file (K-file) and the Hedström file. The shape of a Hedström file is that of inner-stacked cones. Its carrier effect is produced by a straight pull of the file. Hedström files produce a clean, but not cylindrical or smooth, wall. They are best used to cleanse and shape the coronal portion of the canal.

The K-file is similar in design to a reamer, but has a tighter twist and is operated either in a push-and-pull motion or by being rotated clockwise 90° and pulled coronally. It will break easily if lodged tightly in the canal, and also if twisted counterclockwise in an effort to dislodge an embedded file. K-files produce a clean, smooth, cylindrical canal wall and, because of their design, are best used to cleanse and shape the apical portion of the canal.

K-files are stiffer and stronger, size for size, than the Hedström files because of their style of manufacture. To create K-files, a square, rhomboid or triangular rod is twisted, creating cutting flutes. A Hedström file is created when a spiral groove is machined into the rod. It is weaker than a K-file because its central core has been reduced in diameter.

Answer 220

1 A *persistent* deciduous canine tooth on the right maxilla. Although the term *retained* deciduous canine tooth is commonly used for this condition, persistent is correct. 'Retained' refers to failure to erupt, while 'persistent' in this context means failure to exfoliate.

2 In most cases the permanent tooth develops normally, although the time and direction of eruption may be influenced by the persistent deciduous tooth. Persistent deciduous canine teeth may cause linguoversion of the erupting mandibular canine teeth and facial deviation of the maxillary canine teeth (see **136**). Furthermore, persistent deciduous teeth alter the gingival contour, which results in plaque and debris accumulating between the deciduous and permanent teeth.

3 The right maxillary deciduous canine tooth is tooth 504 in the Triadan system (see **225**).

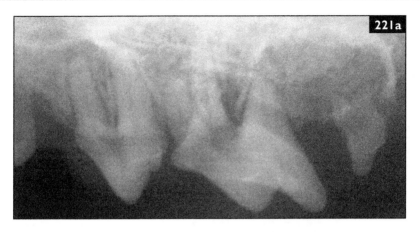

Question 221 This radiograph (**221a**) was obtained using an extraoral technique. Briefly explain this technique.

Question 222 This radiograph (**222**) shows a healing horizontal root fracture of a right maxillary second incisor tooth in a dog.

1 Define crown–root fracture and root fracture.
2 Which type of root fracture offers the best prognosis for maintaining the tooth?
3 What treatment options are available for the different kinds of root fractures?

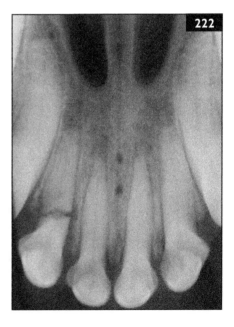

Answer 221 Image overlap of the zygomatic arch and opposite maxillary premolar teeth commonly occurs in the cat. In order to avoid this problem, the extraoral,

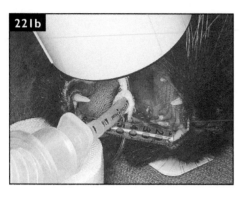

near-parallel technique is recommended (**221b**). With the animal in lateral recumbency, the dental film is placed under the head (under the side which you wish to radiograph) with the mouth propped open. Visualize the central X-ray beam to be perpendicular to the maxillary root axes. Any films used extraorally must be marked to separate them from intraorally exposed film to ensure proper orientation.

Answer 222

1 A crown–root fracture is a fracture involving enamel, dentin, and cementum. These fractures may further be classified as complicated or uncomplicated depending on whether or not the pulp is involved in the fracture line. A root fracture is a fracture involving dentin, cementum, and the pulp, and is generally complicated.

2 The treatment and prognosis of crown and root fractures depends on: (1) the degree of displacement and mobility of the fracture segments; (2) the extent of contamination; and (3) the amount of damage to the alveolar margin bone. Generally, horizontal root fractures involving the apical segment as well as mid-root level respond well to treatment. Fractures of the root close to the gingival margin are unlikely to heal. If the root is to be retained, it will need endodontic therapy.

3 Treatment options depend on the type of fracture. The fracture level determines the choice of treatment for horizontal root fractures. Many fractures involving the apical third of the root heal without treatment, largely because the fracture is stable and the blood supply is intact. The chances of successful healing decrease as the fracture line moves coronally because of the reduced stability. Mid-root fractures usually heal well if the tooth is immobilized using a semi-rigid intraoral composite splint. A horizontal fracture of the coronal part of the root is unlikely to heal. The coronal segment should be extracted and the root treated endodontically if retained. The coronal segment should be removed and the apical segment either extracted or treated endodontically depending on its size.

Question 223
1 Describe the instrument (223a).
2 Which structure is being investigated on this 13-year-old thoroughbred gelding?

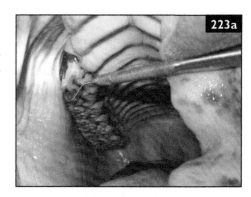

Question 224 This tooth fractured 8 hours ago when the dog tried to catch a rock (224).
1 List two endodontic treatment options for this tooth.
2 What are the advantages and disadvantages of each?

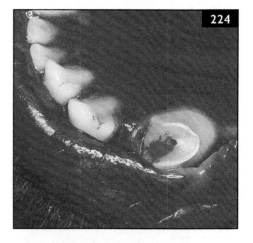

Question 225 This is an intraoral radiograph of an 8-year-old dog (225). The convex surface of the embossed dot is facing the reader.
1 What is the designation of the three-rooted tooth indicated by the arrow, according to the modified Triadan system?
2 What are the advantages of using the Triadan system?
3 What are the disadvantages of using the Triadan system?

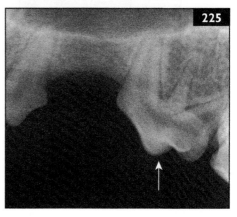

Answer 223

1 The instrument is an extended dental explorer for detecting diseased dentin on the occlusal surface of the horse.

2 The secondary dentin of the pulp horns should be examined visually with a dental mirror and with the explorer to identify any potential exposures of the pulp horns. This figure demonstrates the explorer plunged into pulp horn 2 of the right maxillary second premolar tooth with endodontic disease. The normal occlusal surface of a pulp horn should never allow the tip of the explorer to stick or enter the pulp horn. Each infundibulum normally will have a small central defect left from development where a vessel once entered the structure. Further diagnostics should be performed to determine the vitality of the tooth. Extraoral 30° left dorsal to right ventral oblique radiograph, intraoral bisecting angle technique, or computed tomography are all imaging modalities that can be performed. The normal occlusal anatomy of the maxillary cheek teeth include 2 infundibula and 5 pulp horns. The maxillary second premolar teeth and third molar teeth have additional pulp horns, (second premolar teeth, 6, and third molar teeth, 7). Figure **223b** depicts pulp horn exposure of the left

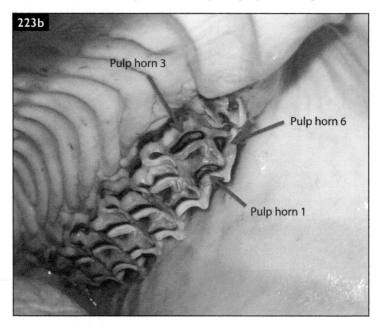

maxillary second premolar tooth. Note the left maxillary first premolar tooth present as well positioned mesially to the second premolar tooth.

Answer 224

1 (1) Standard root canal therapy (total pulpectomy). (2) Vital pulp therapy (partial coronal pulpectomy or pulpotomy).

2 The advantage of standard root canal therapy is its high long-term success rate. One disadvantage of this treatment is that the procedure takes longer, resulting in higher initial costs and longer anesthesia. Also, a non-vital, endodontically treated tooth may be more prone to subsequent fracture. This effect is due mostly to the tooth structure removed during access and canal preparation and also to the tooth becoming more brittle due to the loss of the organic component. Another disadvantage of root canal therapy of an immature tooth is that further maturation and dentin production is arrested.

A vital pulp therapy (partial coronal pulpectomy or pulpotomy) is faster and easier to perform and therefore less costly. If successful, the pulp remains vital. For an immature tooth, this allows the tooth to become stronger as secondary dentin is formed. A partial coronal pulpectomy involves the atraumatic removal of the coronal 2–8 mm of pulp (depending on the size of the tooth), both to eliminate contaminated tissue and to provide space for a restoration. Calcium hydroxide [$Ca(OH)_2$] or mineral trioxide aggregate (MTA) is applied to the exposed pulp, followed by an intermediate layer. Then a final bonded composite restoration is placed.

One disadvantage of a partial coronal pulpectomy is the reported failure rate of 10–20%. If the pulp were contaminated or suffering a traumatic, irreversible pulpitis, the tooth would require full root canal therapy in the future. Vitally treated teeth should be monitored for 5 or 6 years, as failures can occur long after treatment. Pulp vitality testing in animals under clinical circumstances is difficult, and radiography remains the most practical means of follow-up examination.

Answer 225

1 Number 207. It is the left maxillary third premolar tooth, which has a supernumerary root. The second premolar tooth is absent. The Triadan system utilizes a three-digit number to designate each tooth. Quadrants are designated by the first digit and rotate from right maxilla → left maxilla → left mandible → right mandible; the rotation is designated with numbers 1 through 4.

The quadrant numbering continues with numbers 5 through 8 for primary teeth. Each individual tooth has a two-digit designation, beginning with 01 for the first incisor tooth (the one closest to the midline) and continuing in ascending order to the distal end of the arch in each quadrant. In the dog, the last maxillary tooth is normally number 10 and the last mandibular tooth is normally number 11.

The 'Rule of Four and Nine' is used to provide consistency among varying species. The number 04 always designates a canine tooth and the number 09 always designates a first molar tooth. The number normally used for a tooth that is not included in the dental formula of a given species is not used on its chart. For example, in the cat, which normally does not have the maxillary first premolar tooth, the numbers 105 and 205 are not used. This system works for dogs, cats, rodents, pigs, horses, cattle, sheep, etc.

2 (1) The Triadan system is adaptable to computer use. (2) Each tooth has a unique number; there is no confusion when referring to left, right, maxillary, or mandibular teeth. (3) The system is consistent and easy to use with a variety of species, even those with a reduced dentition. (4) It is convenient to use in conjunction with anatomic charts.

3 (1) The Triadan system is difficult to remember if not used on a regular basis. (2) Tooth function and anatomic connotation are not identified by the number.

Question 226 The clinical appearance of dental caries in a dog is shown (226).
1 Define dental caries, and comment on the etiology.
2 Describe the clinical aspects of dental caries in the dog and cat.

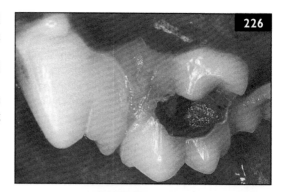

Question 227 Following root canal treatment and placement of an intermediate-layer restoration on this incisor tooth (227):
1 Which restorative material would you choose to restore the access site and why?
2 What are the important characteristics of this material?

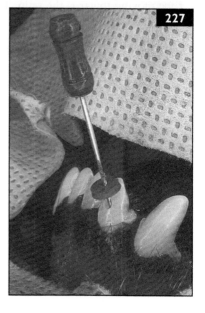

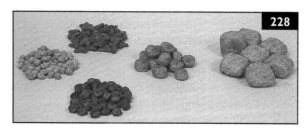

Question 228 How does food texture and composition affect the development of periodontal disease in the dog and cat (228)?

Answer 226

1 In a broad sense, dental caries is defined as a microbial disease of the calcified tissues of the tooth, characterized by demineralization of the inorganic portion and destruction of the organic substance of the tooth. The etiology is complex and there is no consensus on the relative importance of acid-producing bacteria, proteolytic bacteria, and the role of chelation.

2 In dogs, the most common type and site of dental caries is occlusal caries (G.V. Black type I) affecting the mandibular and maxillary molar teeth. The fissured areas of the occlusal surfaces of these teeth provide an ideal harbor for the microorganisms causing caries. Once the dentinoenamel junction is reached, the caries lesion spreads into the dentin, undermining the enamel, while at the same time moving towards the pulp. The undermined enamel may fracture. Inflamed or exposed pulp is associated with pain.

In dogs, the typical early chalky-white, soft lesions are often overlooked. Dental caries is generally diagnosed in an advanced stage: multiple, highly pigmented yellow or brown lesions affecting several (pre)molar teeth with a hard, leathery, or sclerosed surface. As soon as a clinically detectable dental caries lesion has occurred, the choice of treatment is restorative dentistry or extraction, depending on the extent of the lesion.

Cervical dental caries occurs on either buccal, lingual, or interproximal surfaces. In dogs with gingival recession or severe periodontal disease the dental caries process may readily commence in the exposed cementum or dentin (root caries).

True caries in cats is rare; resorptive lesions are a different dental disease.

Answer 227

1 A composite restoration would provide the best esthetics with the least amount of tooth loss.

2 The word composite describes a material which has two constituents which are insoluble in each with a definitive interface between them. Composites contain an organic resin matrix, an inorganic filler, and a coupling agent that bonds the two together. Composites with higher amounts of filler have superior physical and mechanical properties. The major families of composites are traditionally classified by filler size, and include: the microfilled composites, which have a particle size of 0.02–0.04 nm and a lower fill load of 20–55% volume contributing to their lesser strength but good polishability; hybrid composites with a particle size of 0.06–1.0 nm and a 60–65% filler load that imparts greater strength but poorer polishability (matte finish); microhybrids with smaller-size filler particles (0.4 nm) than the hybrid composites, but high, 70–75% by weight, filler content; and the nanofilled composites, which include both nanofilled resins and nanohybrids. Nanofilled resins contain nanofilled particles throughout the resin whereas nanohybrid composites contain nanofilled particles/nanomers (5–75 nm)

in addition to traditional fillers. Both nano subcategories result in composites that rival traditional microhybrids in strength, but have enhanced polishability and retention of surface smoothness. As a general rule, microfilled composites are used only for rostral restorations in the mouth, where esthetics are paramount and high strength is less of a factor, and hybrid composites are used for caudally-located restorations due to their high strength, but not rostrally due to their lesser esthetics, whereas microhybrids and nanohybrids are more of a true universal restorative material that may be used for both rostral and caudal restorations.

Answer 228 Balanced dry dental diets with enhanced textural characteristics (i.e. so-called mechanical dental diets) that do not shatter readily upon tooth contact promote chewing and have improved contact with tooth surfaces, and can be an effective adjunctive method of plaque reduction. To say, however, that any generic dry diet has a dental benefit over soft diets is an overstatement, and is largely unsubstantiated in large epidemiologic studies. Chewing activity and the chewing of harder foods influences salivary flow and the composition of the oral flora, which may in turn impact oral health beyond the favorable mechanical action. No controlled studies exist that compare natural 'raw' food diets against commercial diets to substantiate the claim that dogs and cats consuming a natural diet have less periodontal disease than dogs and cats receiving a commercial pet food. There are reports that show dogs and cats receiving a natural diet have less calculus accumulation, but not necessarily less periodontal disease; pets on a natural diet have an increase in tooth fractures. One should keep in mind that a reduction in dental plaque or calculus by a particular diet may not necessarily directly translate into a defense against or reversal of periodontal disease. Sodium hexametaphosphate (SHMP) is the most common of the chemical anti-calculus food coatings. SHMP is a chelator or sequestrant of salivary calcium, reducing its availability for incorporation with dental plaque to form calculus, and is utilized as a coating for dry diets, baked biscuits and rawhide chews. There are studies that support and others that show no benefit of SHMP in reducing calculus accumulation, but the common denominator is that a high-enough concentration of SHMP must be available, and that SHMP must be used as a coating of the food item, not simply an ingredient in the food, for there to be a positive anti-calculus benefit.

Index

Note: Page references are to question number

Also available in the Self-Assessment Color Review series

Printed and bound by CPI Group (UK) Ltd, Croydon, CR0 4YY

23/10/2024

01777696-0002